Brain Injury, Trauma and Loss

Brain Injury, Trauma and Loss tells the story of the impact of Covid-19 on neurorehabilitation.

It offers a unique dual perspective as it intertwines the two voices of Sue Williams, who had sustained a traumatic brain injury in 2018, and Rudi Coetzer, her neuropsychologist during the pandemic. Based on detailed diary extracts, therapeutic notes and updates (edited to preserve confidentiality), this book provides a unique insight into the practical and psychological effects of Covid-19 on brain injury and rehabilitation, ranging from the impact on delivering clinical rehabilitation sessions and self-directed approaches, to the effect on daily living, social isolation, and online integration. The final section on 'reflections' contributes to the current wider knowledge on how to improve practice in brain injury rehabilitation for patients, families and clinicians. The detailed account of changes in service delivery provides a window into what kind of adaptations can be made in clinical practices, highlighting the need to question existing practices and look for creative methods in delivering rehabilitation services.

This is valuable reading for clinical neuropsychologists who experienced changes in their work both during and since the pandemic, as well as speech therapists, occupational therapists, physiotherapists, and brain injury survivors, their families, and friends.

Sue Williams is a Social-Psychologist and works as an applied researcher in environmental social science for a national government body. Sue sustained a traumatic brain injury in a cycling accident in 2018. She is now actively engaged in brain injury research projects and expert committees.

Rudi Coetzer is a Consultant Neuropsychologist who has worked in senior clinical, academic and leadership roles within the NHS, universities, and charitable sectors of the UK.

After Brain Injury: Survivor Stories

This new series of books is aimed at those who have suffered a brain injury and their families and carers. Each book focuses on a different condition, such as face blindness, amnesia and neglect, or a diagnosis, such as encephalitis and locked-in syndrome, resulting from brain injury. Readers will learn about life before the brain injury, the early days of diagnosis, the effects of the brain injury, the process of rehabilitation, and life now. Alongside this personal perspective, professional commentary is also provided by a specialist in neuropsychological rehabilitation, making the books relevant for professionals working in rehabilitation, such as psychologists, speech and language therapists, occupational therapists, social workers and rehabilitation doctors. They will also appeal to clinical psychology trainees and undergraduate and graduate students in neuropsychology, rehabilitation science, and related courses who value the case study approach.

With this series, we also hope to help expand awareness of brain injury and its consequences. The World Health Organization has recently acknowledged the need to raise the profile of mental health issues (with the WHO Mental Health Action Plan 2013-20) and we believe there needs to be a similar focus on psychological, neurological and behavioural issues caused by brain disorders, and a deeper understanding of the importance of rehabilitation support. Giving a voice to these survivors of brain injury is a step in the right direction.

Series Editor: Barbara A. Wilson

Published titles:

Reconstructing Identity After Brain Injury
A search for hope and optimism after maxillofacial and neurosurgery
Stijn Geerinck

Belonging After Brain Injury
Relocating Dan
Katie H.Williams

Blossoming Into Disability Culture Following Traumatic Brain Injury
The Lotus Arising
Dee Phyllis Genetti

Neuropsychological Consequences of COVID-19
Life After Stroke and Balint's Syndrome
Jwala Narayanan, Anjana Xavier, Jonathan Evans, Narinder Kapur and Barbara Wilson

Brain Injury, Trauma and Loss
Rehabilitation During Covid-19
Sue Williams and Rudi Coetzer

For more information about this series, please visit: www.routledge.com/After-Brain-Injury-Survivor-Stories/book-series/ABI

Brain Injury, Trauma and Loss

Rehabilitation During Covid-19

Sue Williams and Rudi Coetzer

Routledge
Taylor & Francis Group

LONDON AND NEW YORK

Designed cover image: Sue Williams

First published 2026
by Routledge
4 Park Square, Milton Park, Abingdon, Oxon OX14 4RN

and by Routledge
605 Third Avenue, New York, NY 10158

Routledge is an imprint of the Taylor & Francis Group, an informa business

British Library Cataloguing-in-Publication Data
A catalogue record for this book is available from the British Library

ISBN: 9781032833897 (hbk)
ISBN: 9781032827933 (pbk)
ISBN: 9781003509134 (ebk)

DOI: 10.4324/9781003509134

Typeset in Times New Roman
by Newgen Publishing UK

Sue Williams dedication:
In loving memory of Mum and Pete
forever in my heart, always in my mind.

Rudi Coetzer dedication:
For the patients I saw during the pandemic,
and my colleagues who were there, present.

Contents

Introduction

I never expected to have a brain injury. In my occasional musings of potential life events, a traumatic brain injury was never on the agenda. But in August 2018, I was hit by a car whilst out cycling. This devastating accident left me with a brain injury which was absolutely life-changing. Whilst initially I was grateful to still be physically alive, I also slowly and painfully found out that a large part of me had in many ways 'died' on the road on that fateful day. I had changed, in ways far beyond what I could comprehend or manage … a seismic alteration to my psychological sense of 'self', my cognitive abilities, and my interactions with family, friends, work and the wider world around me. On that fateful day in August, I had started as the 'original me' – a 50 year old intelligent professional, passionate about my work as an environmental social scientist, an enthusiastic endurance racing cyclist, a caring sister and daughter, an independent equal partner and a strong advocate for challenging inequality and encouraging participation by all in society. By the end of that day, I had sustained a traumatic brain injury, which would go on to change almost every aspect of my life. A 'new normal' had begun, even though I had little understanding of it at the time.

DOI: 10.4324/9781003509134-1

However, it was not to be the only significant change. In early 2020, none of us expected Covid-19 to come hurtling over the horizon like a viral version of an invading army. Despite the news of an emerging virus, first in China and then in Europe, what was something 'over there' all too soon became 'it's here'. Like everyone else, I was unprepared. Covid-19 changed all of our worlds and we had to manage new ways of living, with lockdowns and social distancing becoming day-to-day events. Another 'new normal' had begun, not just for me but for everyone.

As we continue to move forward in this 'post-pandemic' world there will be many accounts of the impact of Covid-19, along with increasing research on the effect that it had on individuals with a brain injury, rehabilitation, and within the NHS. However, these are often written as objective research papers based on the results of clinical studies, social surveys, and qualitative interviews by academics and clinicians. Although robust and useful, these studies 'speak for' others, and in doing so can lose the powerful insights of a more direct voice.

This book offers a different insight. The interwoven stories of two people, based on the lived experiences of a neuropsychologist (Rudi) and myself, Sue, a brain injury survivor who was just starting rehabilitation and trying to cope with the challenging consequences. In many ways, it provides a detailed account from both sides of the (virtual) desk and, in doing so, illustrates how change affects all of us. No-one was an 'expert' when it came to managing the day-to-day immediate impacts of Covid-19 on us all, personally and professionally.

The following chapters provide not only a vivid account of our respective lived experiences during Covid-19, but also pose a number of fundamental questions. What difference did it make having a brain injury during Covid-19? What effect did the virus have on neurorehabilitation? How much change can an individual cope with simultaneously? How did we manage the mental health impacts of the pandemic? What was the effect of the pandemic on the NHS and the dedicated staff who had to immediately step up to cope with a global medical emergency? The following chapters address these questions, and more, through our personal accounts of our lived experiences during the pandemic.

Like all good stories, this book has a beginning and a middle, although the 'end' is still on-going as I continue to live with a brain injury and we all now adjust to a life with Covid-19. However, in this book there are also two 'new beginnings' – the first originating from the day of my accident when I sustained a traumatic brain injury, and the second at the start of the pandemic in the UK in early 2020. Part 1 of this book describes my accident and the initial 18 months of my brain injury before Covid-19 reared its head. Part 2 of this book covers life during the most disruptive years of the pandemic, as rapid change and psychological adjustment was required in the context of an unknown virus that swept the world. It explores the impact of these tumultuous years through the stories of both myself and Rudi as we experienced various challenges and issues during the time. The final part of the book reflects on these experiences, and considers the overall changes and impacts from this unique period as we move forward into the future.

Although there is no final end to this story, there are reflections and insights from this shared experience. Hopefully, from these we can all understand more about the effect of having a brain injury, the changes that happen, and the impact that has on both the individual and their family and friends. It also shines a light on the real-world experiences of the valued staff in the NHS who rose admirably to the challenge of the pandemic, providing much-needed critical care during an unprecedented time.

Part 1

Before Covid-19

Chapter 1

Traumatic Brain Injury

Sue Williams and Rudi Coetzer

(i) The Beginning and the End

Saturday August 11, 2018 – Time to Ride!

I remember that morning so clearly. As with every Saturday, my alarm had gone off at 7am, and I was up, showered and out – cycling kit on, big breakfast eaten and bike checked. A standard routine of most weekends was to join the regular 'club ride' that met at 9am every Saturday near my house in North Wales. I'd been riding with the cycling club for years, and absolutely loved it. I really enjoyed the challenge of a hard, hilly, 100 mile 'century ride', the banter between riders, the freedom to explore the quiet lanes and climbs around the mountains of Snowdonia – not forgetting the all-important mid-ride café stop.

It was a good day for cycling – warm, dry, no wind or rain. I was absolutely pinging, bursting with energy, feeling fit and fast. I'd recently returned from an amazing three weeks in the alps, cycling daily up the biggest, hardest mountain climbs. I'd had a fantastic time, flying up the climbs past glaciers and snow fields listening to the call of the alpine marmots. I knew I was 'cycling fit' after years of training and racing in the Alps, Dolomites and Pyrenees, where the long mountain climbs suited

DOI: 10.4324/9781003509134-3

my lightweight-endurance abilities. Now I was back in Wales and looking forward to meeting up with the cycling club again for a more chilled out ride with my friends.

As usual I'd suggested a hard, fast ride with lots of steep climbs, but only one young rider wanted to come along! The rest of the club wanted a more moderate 70- mile ride – still hilly and long, but at a more sociable pace. For once I wanted to chat with friends more than I wanted to push myself hard on my bike, so I joined forces with the main club ride. It was a great ride, with quiet back roads, empty moorlands and lots of time to chat and catch up with everyone. The group split mid-ride and I formed a small 'advance posse' which went ahead to the café. After the requisite tea and beans on toast, six of us decided to head back over the mountains and return home. It was a steady pace, relaxed, easy, sociable. A normal, everyday ride.

On the final stretch, ten minutes from my house, on our usual quiet back lane, everything changed. From this point on, my life would never be the same again.

CAR! RED CAR! DANGER!
   It's filling the road, it's all I can see, the car looms larger and larger in front of me.
   It's straight ahead, I know I can't get around it...

BRAKE ... BRAKE ...
   I'm gripping the brakes, so hard I can feel the bike shuddering, I'm pushing down on the ped-als, I know I can't stop in time, I'm going to hit it, I can't escape, the car is all there, is in front of me, so big it fills my vision and there is nothing else to

see. A few split seconds feels like an eternity with the awful awareness of death facing me.

CAR ... RED CAR ... IMPACT
DARKNESS
NOTHING
I AM GONE
There is nothing, I don't exist, I am gone. I don't know where. There is no sense of time or place, or even of time passing, no existence. The world has disappeared along with me. Just a total absence of anything. No sight, no sound. Nothing.

PAIN
My head ... agonising ... a ball of pain ... hot, burning pain ...
BLOOD and BONE
Blood ... thick, viscous blood ... filling my mouth ...
sharp edges of broken teeth and bone against my tongue ...
my head an agonising ball of hot pain ...
it is too much ... I cannot stay ...
I let go and fall back into the darkness again

DROWNING IN BLOOD
Thick blood is filling my throat. I'm drowning in my own blood.
I struggle to resurface, to stay alive.
I can't hang on; I'm going to die
Terror ... Panic ... Desperation

SENSELESS

Fragments of occasional consciousness, but I am without my senses.

I have no sight – it does not feel that I have my eyes closed, it does not feel that it is dark. It is a complete absence of anything visual. I have no sight at all, I cannot see anything, it is not dark or light, there is no flicker of movement, it is like my sight has completely gone. Nothing exists out there.

I have no feeling of any part of my body below my head. I don't know what position I am in, I can't feel my legs, my arms. I don't know if I am paralysed. I don't know if I still have all the parts of my body, it just does not exist.

My perception of space has gone, I have no awareness of where I am, what is around me, no idea of people, or movement, or sound, or vision or touch. The rest of the world around me has completely disappeared.

The only thing that exists is the ball of pain in my head, the thick viscous blood, the fragments of teeth. The agonising pain is too much … I disappear back into the dark depths of nothingness; I cannot bear to stay in the world when I'm in this much pain.

VOICES

Fragments, only two voices, close by my head – cycling friends – they tug me out of the nothingness. But the pain is too much, I want them to leave me alone, I don't want to come back to life; it's too much for me.

'Stay with us Sue'.
'Breathe'.
'Squeeze my hand if you can hear us'.
Repeat and repeat .. but I can't respond. I'm trying, but my arm and hand don't exist and I can't get any response. Finally, one finger, my middle finger on my right hand can twitch a little. He feels it. I can communicate. But relief is short-lived.

MY THROAT SWELLS.
I CAN NOT BREATHE!
I CAN NOT SPEAK.
PANIC! … TERROR!
I'M GOING TO DIE!
HELP ME!
My throat starts swelling inside. I'm struggling, struggling to breathe, it's getting worse. But no-one can see it, it's inside, I can't speak, I can't tell anyone. They don't know. I'm trapped inside myself. Panic, terror and fear increasing. I'm going to die as I can't breathe. Help! Please someone help me!

There's a paramedic near my head – I don't know who or where or how long they have been there. I still can't see. I don't know what is going on around me. He's trying to put something on my face, an oxygen mask. But it's making it worse! He doesn't know that I can't breathe! The mask is going to suffocate me!

My arm, I have only one arm that I can feel. I try and try to move it. I'm trying to indicate my throat with my arm. I'm desperate. Please notice! Please help!

The paramedic sees. I think he understands. I hear snippets: 'Code Red'.
Relief. I'm going to live. I let go and disappear back into the pain-free darkness of unconscious-ness again.

I have virtually no memory of what happened immedi-ately after the accident or at the hospital. In fact much of my memory was very patchy even for weeks after-wards. So most of my knowledge has come from others who have subsequently described things to me. My friends had called my partner Mike immediately and he had dashed to the scene to find me semi-conscious, bleeding and unable to respond, lying on the road sur-rounded by paramedics. It was obviously extremely dis-tressing for him, although I was completely unaware of all this at the time. I was placed in an inflatable full body stretcher, my head and neck strapped between blocks. Still mostly unconscious and in pain, I was rushed off in the ambulance as a 'code red' emergency to the Major Trauma Unit at Accident and Emergency.

When Mike arrived at the hospital he was told by the Trauma Consultant that they hoped I would survive, but there were many considerations regarding possible spinal and brain injuries. Mike told me afterwards how utterly shocked he was at this news, he had no idea at the time that my life had been hanging in the balance. Apparently I had various computed tomography (CT) scans and there were many specialists studying my results, con-cerned about paralysis, followed by numerous tests by consultants in the trauma team. I have no recollection of these things. My only memories are isolated, fragmented images of brief moments – the white ceiling tiles as I was being pushed down a corridor, the kind face of a nurse bending over me, the pain of a catheter and the gag reflex of a camera down my throat.

Time had no meaning for me, but eventually I was considered stable enough to go from the major trauma unit to a surgical ward in the hospital. The following day, I had extensive surgery on my badly broken jaw bone and displaced teeth. I recall coming round from hours of surgery to the agony of an incredibly painful trachea, worsened by the oxygen mask strapped on my face. However, after a while the benefits of intravenous morphine meant that I did not feel as bad as I actually was, and Mike arrived to visit to find me relatively chipper. I remember thinking to myself in my hospital bed, attached to various machines and drips, that I would soon be back on my bike and would still be able to do the races I had planned for September. How mistaken that assumption was proven to be!

At the time, no-one had actually mentioned the word 'brain injury' to me. I had slipped through the diagnosis net at the hospital. When I was discharged from the hospital, my partner was told to 'keep an eye on me for 48 hours' in case of concussion. Little did we know at that point that my brain injury would mean that he would be keeping a watch over me for far longer than that and would continue to provide support for the next five years.

(ii) What's Happened to Me?

The first few weeks passed in a blur. I still have limited memories of this time, but apparently I spent most of the time sleeping, with occasional attempts to eat. I had been told by the hospital that I would be on a 'liquid only' diet for several months whilst my jaw and teeth healed. I couldn't open my mouth and was in much pain, so unsurprisingly, eating was extremely difficult. I rapidly lost a dangerous amount of weight, especially as, at that time, I was very thin due to cycle racing and didn't have any spare fat to lose. Fortunately, the dieticians from the hospital came to the rescue, and sent me a regular delivery of liquid medical replacement milkshakes – rather sickly but necessary.

I was surprised to find that I had also lost my sense of smell and my taste had changed completely. Nothing seemed the same, and things I used to like were now repulsive. Little did I know at the time that this was due to the damage in my brain. After a few weeks it also became apparent that my utter debilitating exhaustion and constant sleeping was more significant than 'concussion'. Whilst I expected my head to hurt given the impact, I could sense inside myself that 'something' was fundamentally wrong in my brain. I couldn't find words to describe this sensation, and it wasn't something that anyone could see, but it was definitely an incontrovertible feeling. I was no longer 'me' in a very strange and scary way. I felt so vulnerable, fragile and self-protective.

To begin with I tried to rest as much as possible and was signed off work for six months. I would lie on the sofa for days trying to watch boring daytime TV or to read. But I soon found that I couldn't read more than one sentence, nor follow even the most trivial of TV programmes. I still couldn't speak due to the damage to my jaw and teeth, so had to resort to writing notes.

This was equally difficult and conversation was virtually impossible. Worst of all, I found that I couldn't bear light, whether that was from the sun or a lamp. I kept the curtains closed and spent most of the day in the dark. Sounds and movement were also unbearably painful, so I frequently shut myself away in my room.

After a month – I remember it was a lovely sunny day – I thought I would try to sit in the garden. Mike put a chair out on the patio and I shuffled over. Sitting, I lifted my face to the sun, but the pain in my brain was unbearable. Even the feeling of a gentle breeze on my skin felt too much to bear. With immense sadness, I shuffled back inside. Looking out of the window from my lounge, I saw my local moors bathed in golden light. Slowly tears rolled down my cheeks, as I wondered if I would ever be able to get back up into my beloved mountains again.

Physically, many of my injuries slowly started to heal over the following months. Mike had temporarily moved into my house to look after me, but I wanted to be independent again so asked him to return to his home and just visit every day instead. My closest friends rallied around when I first tried to emerge, acting as my 'bimble buddies' when the most I could manage was a short shuffle to a bench. Slowly I got a bit more used to daylight, although flickering sunlight remains unbearable to me even today. However, noise, conversations and movement were extremely distressing, and I continued to hide away as much as possible.

I knew that there was something going very wrong in my brain. I had significant memory problems, word-finding difficulties and overwhelming fatigue. I got easily confused, and would go around and around in circles in my head about even the most simple things. Trying to leave the house was an exhausting process. I would have to take my keys, wallet and phone, but as soon as I put one of them in my coat pocket, I would no longer remember if I had put it there. I'd check again for my phone, and then worry if I had missed my keys, over and over again. I tried writing post-it note reminders and sticking them to the front door, but it didn't really make the process any easier. As soon as I seemed to do something, I could not recall if I had done it, and the worry and panic would set in.

Debilitating fatigue would often hit me at unexpected times. I would try to go for a little stroll, but part way round, overwhelming exhaustion would come over me like a tidal wave. I'd try to hang on and often wondered if I would be able to make it home. Sometimes I couldn't continue and I would suddenly keel over and curl up in a ball on the ground, my eyes closed and my fingers in my ears to cut out all the light and sound. Mike would do his best to protect and support me, sitting silently beside me and trying to keep other people away. This must have been so difficult for him. Neither of us knew anything about brain injuries at this point, we had no support and were just trying to cope as best as we could with all these strange and disturbing experiences.

Reading continued to be impossible for me which, as an academic and veritable bookworm, I found incredibly distressing. Even though my jaw had healed enough for me to be able to speak, I still found talking difficult. I struggled with the 'flow' of speaking, often losing my words and repeatedly saying 'um'. If I persevered this would get worse and my brain would start crashing, ultimately rendering me incapable of talking at all. Conversations would be frequently unbearable, especially if they went on for even a minute too long. My brain would feel like it was swelling, and the pain would be agonising. I couldn't concentrate on what was being said, and it took everything I had to just not slam down the phone or flee the room. I would silently scream in my head 'shut up, stop now' as someone would try to carry on a normal conversation, biting my lip and trying not to say it out loud in a fit of painful rage.

I found some visual things very confusing; usually anything that looked the same, such as railings or road bollards, or even a row of identical tree trunks. My brain would just seize, it seemed to not be able to make sense of these things that looked the same, and in response my body would freeze. The only way I could manage to move would be to close my eyes, hold Mike's hand and let him guide me through. The worst experiences were when I felt I had been suddenly teleported into a different reality. I would be out and look around me, with absolutely no idea where I was or how to get home. Part of me knew I must have got myself there, but I did not recognise anything. It was utterly terrifying. Was I completely losing my mind?

Despite these significantly distressing symptoms, I tried to pretend that I could manage to still do some things. Unsurprisingly, this went badly wrong over and over again. When I eventually tried to return to work after six months, my attempts pushed me beyond my limits and I ended up in some risky situations. Despite the support of my manager and colleagues, it was far too much for me, and I fell further and further behind. I even tried to go cycling again, but this would inevitably end up with me collapsing mid-ride. I would stagger off my bike and hide, curled up in a semi-comatose ball in a field behind a hedge so that no-one could see me. I desperately wanted to go back to my old life and firmly believed that if I just pushed myself harder I would be able to do it. It didn't help that sometimes I could do some things, so then I would wonder 'am I a fraud?' But inevitably I had to accept that I couldn't cope and that there was something fundamentally wrong with my brain. Little did I know at this point that it would be the start of the longest, hardest journey of my life.

Chapter 2

Accessing Rehab

Sue Williams and Rudi Coetzer

(i) I Need Some Help

As with many people with a brain injury, my rehabilitation journey has not been straightforward nor always timely. Even prior to the massive disruption of the pandemic, there were issues and challenges regarding access to appropriate specialist expertise. I'm not alone in this challenge of accessing support. Although each experience is unique to the individual, my experience illustrates some shared issues and, more importantly, also describes how that feels, along with the impact this has on the individual and their families, work and social activities, both psychologically and practically.

Increasingly, there have been calls for improvements to patients' access to appropriate diagnosis and rehabilitation. The National Neurosciences Advisory Group (NNAG) has recently published the 'Optimal Clinical Pathway for Adults: Traumatic Brain Injury' (NNAG, 2023). This focuses on the importance of providing an 'integrated care pathway' which brings together all the elements from acute to long-term rehabilitation. The need for improvement is highlighted by a review of the current lack of an appropriate service, with the NNAG stating that this leads to mis-diagnosis (or, as in my

DOI: 10.4324/9781003509134-4

case, no diagnosis initially), along with poor rehabilitation outcomes and, worse, long-term disability.

This optimised clinical pathway for people with a traumatic brain injury (TBI) aims to integrate A&E, GPs, local neurology services and regional centres. Integral to this, the role of a 'first point of contact' or 'case manager' has been highlighted as being of particular importance to patients. Having a single trusted person, who is experienced in supporting a person with a brain injury, from the initial point of injury through an often prolonged period of rehabilitation, would have meant a great deal to me. Unfortunately that wasn't my experience; although, at a later stage in my rehab journey, I really appreciated coming under the care of the North Wales Brain Injury Service in the NHS, which provided me with much needed continuity.

Whilst the 'Optimised Clinical Pathway' is an example of best practice, the reality faced by most of us with a traumatic brain injury is far from this. Rather than a seamless pathway, guided and supported by a trusted professional, my experience was initially more of trying to access a fractured, confusing and challenging system, which was difficult to understand and navigate. What made this even harder for someone like me with a traumatic brain injury was that I had additional injuries and psychological issues. This increased the number of different areas of the medical system that I had to try to manage and co-ordinate at a time when I was struggling significantly with the effects of executive dysfunction which made planning, remembering and attending multiple appointments very challenging. It was also a system about which I had very little pre-existing knowledge, so having to suddenly learn and understand 'who does what' was very cognitively demanding. There appeared to be little recognition across the diversity of different hospital departments of the issues faced by someone like me who also had a brain injury. As my partner said when he looked at my calendar and the myriad of appointment letters from different consultants pinned to my board, 'keeping on top of this would be hard enough without a brain injury, how on earth are you expected to manage with a brain injury?' All too often there was an assumption that there would be a family member available to help me, regardless of whether or not that was the case. As someone who lived alone and valued their independence, I was determined to try to cope and the expectation that I would be dependent on someone else was another way of eroding my self-identity.

It is difficult to pinpoint exactly when my 'rehab' began, or even when I got a specific diagnosis of having a brain injury. Rather than a clear event, it was more of a drawn-out confusing process. As described in the preceding chapter, my head-first collision with a car caused substantial trauma as my soft brain ricocheted backwards and forwards in the hard bony case of my skull. Despite this, the hospital did not mention 'traumatic brain injury' – possibly because a CT scan had not shown any bleed on the brain. Leaving the hospital, my only information related to managing on a 'liquid diet' due to my facial injuries and a requirement for 'someone to be with me for 48 hours'. This was due to possible concussion and post-anaesthetic implications following surgery to repair my jawbone and teeth.

Yet, I knew instinctively that something was profoundly 'wrong' in me, I just didn't understand what it was, nor why I was having such conflicting and confusing symptoms. The previous chapter describes these experiences, along with the impact this had on my relationships with my partner, family and friends, and about how the lack of an initial clear diagnosis nor any specific early rehabilitation meant that I tried to return to work, along with attempting to go back to my previous social activities, including cycling. In the absence of knowing what was wrong with me, I tried to just go 'back to normal' even though it really wasn't the right thing for me.

Critical during this period was my local GP. I will remain forever grateful for her support and understanding during this first year after my accident. Like many of us, my first point of contact when something is 'wrong' was my GP. Arriving at her office a few weeks after leaving the hospital, I wobbled up the stairs and tried to explain to her that I thought there was something quite significantly wrong with me. Muddling my words, overwhelmed with fatigue, my GP soon realised over the next few months that I didn't have 'just' temporary concussion. This was the start of a partnership approach between myself and my GP, and I was grateful for both her time and expertise, along with the respect she always showed by listening to my insights about what was happening to me. She also provided a much-needed 'check' to my impatience to return to work. For months I would go for my regular appointment with my GP, feeling convinced that I was more than capable of going back to work. Following a long discussion, where we talked about my continuing fatigue and cognitive problems, I would leave the surgery holding yet another 'sick note' saying I was still not fit to return to work. Disappointed, dejected, feeling worthless, but not knowing what to do about it, I went home to continue alternating between 'doing nothing' and 'overdoing things'.

My GP was also essential in referring me to the North Wales Brain Injury Service for assessment and potential treatment. At the time, there was a requirement for GPs to wait at least six months before being able to refer people with a suspected neurological condition to this specialist brain injury service. It is completely valid to wait to see if a person regains function as a process of natural recovery during these first few months, as well as the practicalities for the NHS of managing overwhelming demand. However, I found it extremely challenging during this period to have no understanding about all the disturbing and confusing symptoms that I was experiencing, nor any advice about how to manage everything.

My experience of a lack of specialist neurological information, diagnosis and follow-up following my accident, especially from the hospital, appears to be similar for many with a traumatic brain injury. A review in The Lancet Neurology on 'Traumatic Brain Injury: progress and challenges in prevention, clinical care, and research' (Maas et al., 2022) highlighted this issue:

Around 50% of adult patients with mild TBI presenting to hospital do not recover to pre-TBI levels of health by six months after their injury. Fewer than 10% of patients discharged after presenting to an emergency department for TBI in Europe currently receive follow-up. Structured follow-up after mild TBI should be considered good practice, and urgent research is needed to identify which patients with mild TBI are at risk for incomplete recovery.

(Maas et al., 2022)

In addition to the potential for delayed or incomplete recovery, those early months were some of the most distressing and challenging for someone like myself who was finally assessed as having a 'moderate' brain injury (traumatic brain injury is generally defined in its simplest terms as 'mild', 'moderate', and 'severe', with even a 'mild' brain injury causing significant difficulties). To suddenly feel like something drastic and disturbing is happening to you, which you don't understand, nor do you know how to respond to, left me scared and confused. To face this alone, without experienced or knowledgeable clinical support, was really difficult. In the absence of knowledge, not only did I not 'improve' but in trying to return to previous activities I put myself at risk and left myself open to greater harm.

The urge to 'return to normal' is probably a strong driver for all of us. I assumed in those first 12 months that I would just 'get better'. I found it so confusing. At times I felt like I could do normal things again, but then when I tried I'd end up with what I called my 'scrambled egg brain', along with overwhelming pain and fatigue. I was still a very long way off understanding the variable nature of my brain injury symptoms, and how I could do some complex tasks but couldn't do other much easier things. Nor did I understand how I might be able to do something first thing in the morning, but by 10am, I couldn't do anything. This lack of knowledge and understanding about the variable effects of my brain injury left me feeling like a fraud. A feeling which was exacerbated by everyone telling me I looked great, and that it didn't look like there was anything wrong with me. Much as I appreciated not looking awful, these comments conflicted with how I was feeling inside and the difficulties I was facing. Maybe I needed to try harder? Maybe I was making it up? After all, if it was really significant surely someone would have said something at the hospital and stepped in to help me?

It is really difficult to explain the inner conflict that I felt between my disturbing experiences, pain and fatigue, compared to how I 'appeared' to my friends, and the lack of any diagnosis of a brain injury. I asked my partner, Mike, about his thoughts of me in the initial stages as he was the only person who was with me in those early days.

> You had changed, immediately. Most of all your confidence had gone. I remember going for a walk, and you gripped my hand so tightly I thought you would cut off my circulation. You were scared, not just of cars, but of everything.
>
> (Mike)

I tried to hide my symptoms – they were too scary; I didn't understand what was happening and I wondered if I had quite literally 'lost my mind'. From my experience, I feel that the psychological impact of not providing appropriate information as early as possible for people with a traumatic brain injury is significantly under-estimated. This period of unexplained symptoms and confusion is surely the time for clinicians to step in with at least some information and support, even if formal assessment and diagnosis need to wait to a later stage.

(ii) Assessments and Tests

Sue's Journal April 2019

It's been eight months since my accident, and my brain hasn't functioned properly since then. I'm on my way to Liverpool, stomach churning, hands sweating, for an appointment with a private consultant neuropsychologist for cognitive tests, as required by the insurance company. My anxiety and stress are driven by a complex mix of uncertainty about what these tests might involve, combined with how I might perform and the impact of the results.

I have no idea what these tests consist of or what I might have to do, and I have little idea about cognition or brain function. I've spent the last few weeks trying to find out, searching the internet for specific details. Although there are many references to cognitive testing, I can't find the actual details of any of these tests.

Why does it matter? After all, like most of us, I have had various medical tests – regular blood tests and occasional scans – and I haven't previously felt the need to know a lot about the procedure. I had a CT scan of my brain in the hospital trauma unit after my accident, but as I have no recollection of that actually happening, I don't remember experiencing any anxiety about either the procedure or the results (actually I have no memory of even knowing the results).

This is different, it's a test, a test of my cognitive functions. It feels more akin to a driving test or a school exam, but without any knowledge of what might be involved and consequently unable to prepare. I feel like I'm going in blind to a test of overwhelming importance.

Sat in a quiet office in the centre of the city; a stranger in a suit in front of me. The assessment began with lots of questions about my life, both before and after my accident. I am as honest as I can be, but there is so much that I can't say. So many disturbing things that are happening with my brain, that I'm too scared to admit, that I keep hidden from everyone. Those moments when I have no idea where I am, when nothing looks familiar and I am scared I won't find my way home. The gaps in my memory, the tidal wave of overwhelming fatigue that leaves me unable to move. The confusion inside my head, and the overwhelming pain of lights and sounds. There are many of these instances that I can't explain and keep locked up inside me, but which are also counterbalanced by the confusion of sometimes feeling almost 'normal' again. Is there really anything wrong with my brain or not?

The tests begin; the neuropsychologist sits opposite me across from the desk with what feels like a never-ending folder of test after test. My anxiety subsides as I focus on each specific task, concentrating hard. I've always been performance-focused, and it is inherent in me to always push myself and do my best. I'm surprised, many of these tasks seem relatively straightforward, and I have a growing feeling that maybe there is nothing wrong with my brain after all.

Then midway through the tests it hits me; the next task, it should be easy, I remember doing this type of thing when I was a child, but I can't, I just can't. I try, I try again. Each time, I know instinctively that I should be able to do this, but I can't. Something is missing in my brain. I don't know what that something is, but it's gone. It felt like reaching into your familiar toolkit, to get the tool you always use, only to find that it's gone, and no matter how hard you search, it's not there. It is impossible to find the words to explain how it feels to suddenly realise that there is something missing in your brain.

I will always remember that moment; it pierced my heart. For the first time, the inescapable, incontrovertible knowledge there was something actually wrong with my brain. I wasn't making it up, it wasn't that I didn't try hard enough, it wasn't just that I'd 'forgotten' things. Some cognitive function in my brain that should have been there had gone. Shaken, I continued; some tests were still straight forward, but others had the same impact when I realised that I wasn't able to do them. On other tasks, I knew I was probably slow, but my brain was straining and I had to check, and check again, each time not quite remembering what had happened the first time. I was exhausted when I finally finished, but more than tired, I was emotionally confused and scared.

Back home, I waited for the report of my test results to arrive. What would it say? It felt like an impossible 'lose-lose' situation. If the tests showed that there was really something wrong with my brain, that filled me with fear and distress. The words 'brain damage' loomed large, and I tried my best to push it to one side. On the other hand, if the tests showed that there was nothing wrong with my brain, then what on earth was causing all these painful, distressing and confusing experiences? Was I going mad? Was I making it up?

Opening up the email and reading the report of my test results was incredibly distressing and stressful. Alone, my hands shaking on the keyboard, I slowly read through an extensive report. There was so much detail, it was hard to process and understand. This was describing 'me' in such clinical and objective terms that I felt like a specimen in a scientific experiment. Whilst many results indicated that I had retained much of my 'premorbid' ability, there were a number of areas where my brain had clearly sustained damage resulting in loss of cognitive functions. My pre-accident capabilities had been referenced as being in the 'Superior Range', consistent with my level of education and occupation as a researcher. However, now in bold type, I read the words 'Low Average' and 'Extremely Low Range' in reference to my working memory and speed of processing, along with a whole new world of terminology relating to cognitive functions and percentiles, most of which I didn't really understand.

As an academic and an applied researcher, it was distressing to read this report, to know there were aspects of my cognitive function that were significantly impaired. It hit hard at the core of my self-identity and professional capability. Although it presented my test results, it didn't address the issues of greatest concern to me. Would I ever get better? What does this mean for my life? Will I still be able to work? Could I go back to enjoying spending time with my friends and family?

It was also hard reading the report with no-one there to answer my questions or to provide appropriately informed reassurance. It came with the realisation that cognitive testing is more akin to an instrument to help inform the start of a process of knowledge and understanding, and the results could not on their own provide an adequate response to the complexity of traumatic brain injury.

Whilst much has been written in the clinical literature about the validity and robustness of cognitive testing, there has been comparatively little research on the lived experience of people with a brain injury undergoing this process. However, a qualitative study of people who have had a Stroke provides insight into the diverse lived experiences of cognitive tests and assessments, and emphasises the lack of research in this area, despite the increasing importance of understanding patient perspectives to improve clinical practice (Hobden et al., 2023). Similar to my experience, Hobden et al.'s (2023) study of cognitive testing divides people's experiences into three areas: (i) before, (ii) during and (iii) after the assessment. It notes the commonality that people feel about the lack of information about tests and their purpose prior to the assessment, along with issues with the use of clinical terminology in post-assessment feedback, with some resorting to trying to find out the definitions of cognitive functions themselves. As with many areas relating to neurological conditions, the study found that people's emotional responses to testing were very diverse, with some experiencing 'test anxiety' similar to myself. This is also reflected in a similar study of the perceptions of people with multiple sclerosis (MS) (Elwick et al., 2022) which found that cognitive assessments have the potential to provoke intense emotions, eliciting feelings of shame and irritation among some patients.

The study of the experience of people who have had a Stroke also noted that anxiety relating to testing was partly linked to an individuals' awareness of their cognitive impairments. It emphasised the importance of providing feedback in a supportive manner due to the impact this can have on an individuals' self-confidence. Although it is important to identify and explain cognitive difficulties, this should also be discussed in the context of an individuals' relative cognitive strengths.

(iii) Neurorehabilitation Begins

Fortunately, my subsequent experience of assessment was much more 'patient friendly' with the support of the NHS. Following my GP referral, in September 2019, I had an initial assessment with a consultant neurologist who referred me to his colleague, Rudi. Rudi was a consultant neuropsychologist and Head of Service at the North Wales Brain Injury Service at the time. So, in November, I sat in the hospital unit waiting for my first session, not knowing what to expect.

Sue's Journal November 2019
'When I tap the pen against the desk, I just want you to say "tap" in response when you hear it' – a simple instruction from the quiet man who sat next to me in a small office in the brain injury unit.

This didn't seem too onerous a task, but as soon as I started, I felt it … the 'stutter' in my brain between hearing and my response. It was impossible to explain this sensation of delay, but it felt like a message wasn't getting through clearly, a break in the connection in my brain. Something wasn't right, but maybe I was just making it up, or being over-sensitive? Surely no-one else will notice this? 'Sound … brain stutter … word' – it just wasn't as seamless and automatic as it used to be. It felt like there was some 'friction in the system' in my brain.

As cognitive testing goes, this was certainly not as stressful or exhausting as my previous experience, but as before, I instinctively knew that something was 'wrong'. The difference was that, in this instance, I was in a situation where I felt that I could ask questions as well as be tested. As part of a thorough assessment, I had been asked about my life before my accident – my education, employment, hobbies and activities, family and friends. Knowing that I had explained my background, I felt for the first time that I could ask why I was able to remember research papers from 20 years ago, but I couldn't leave the house without going round in circles trying to recall if I had put my keys in my pocket. Am I a fraud? Am I making this up? Am I not trying hard enough? Why can I do some things and not other things?

Those initial questions came tumbling out in that first assessment. I was grateful to not be frowned at for wasting Rudi's time, but instead received a reassuring reply. It was apparently to be expected with my type of brain injury that I would retain knowledge of some things that were embedded in my mind from previous extensive use and experience, but the impairment of my working memory was making it hard for my brain to recall new, everyday things that were only being held in my mind for a short period of time. Like pieces in a jigsaw, for the first time I started to see a connection between some of the incomprehensible results of the cognitive testing and the difficulties I was having with everyday life.

So where do I go from here? At least there seemed to be confirmation that there was something wrong with my brain, but I didn't know what would happen next. I hoped that this appointment was not a 'one off', but I wasn't sure if I was going to be sent away with just some information and still no idea about what to do about it all. Could my brain not be fixed in some other way, maybe through medication or by practicing a specific memory task?

In November 2019, it had been over a year since my accident and I was struggling significantly with the effects of my brain injury. Previous approaches of trying to 'fix myself' by just resting followed by a period of pushing hard and attempting to get back to normal had clearly not worked and I felt more overloaded, confused and fatigued than before. I was, therefore, relieved in some ways to be told that this was the start of a process of rehabilitation and I would be coming back for a weekly appointment with Rudi who was to become an integral part of my journey, both in those early stages and during the unexpected Covid-19 pandemic.

However, inside I felt so guilty and ashamed about needing support and taking up such limited NHS resources. This feeling would multiply during the pandemic, knowing how overstretched every single person was within the health service, and how much they were all having to do to cope with the arrival of this new virus. Also, having grown up with a severely disabled brother who faced incredible challenges both physically and cognitively, whilst being cared for every day by my mother, I was painfully aware that there are so many other people who have much greater difficulties than me. Embedded within that shame was a core of my identity that shouted loudly that I was meant to be strong, capable and able to sort my problems out myself. I was someone who helped others, not a person who needed support. It would take me a long time, and a lot of rehab and self-reflection to understand how difficult it is to accept our vulnerabilities, and to see that asking for help is one of the hardest things to do, requiring greater strength and courage than I had ever had to have before.

One of the key questions about the impact of the pandemic on brain injury rehabilitation is whether it made a difference to engage 'in-person' or 'online'. In order to respond to that issue, it is worth reflecting on a few aspects of my experience of in-person appointments at the dedicated North Wales Brain Injury Service.

On the one hand, travelling to places and being in meeting rooms was really challenging for me and caused significant problems relating to cognitive overload as detailed in the previous chapter. However, there were some things about the brain injury unit that immediately helped and were different from other places – the room always felt peaceful and slightly soothing. As someone who had significant difficulties with background noise, other conversations, and flickering lights, the overall 'ambience' of the brain injury unit didn't overload my brain. Having what felt like a more neurologically comfortable space lowered my cognitive load, and consequently reduced my anxiety about appearing to 'embarrass myself' when things got too much for me and I struggled to speak or manage my emotions. There were a few aspects that were unavoidably difficult, such as driving and parking, and the occasional sound of typing in the waiting room, but overall, these disruptions were kept to a minimum.

Positioning was also important, having the space to sit beside someone rather than in front of them or from behind a desk also helped by being less 'in your face'. There is something about being side-by-side that invokes a sense of partnership rather than hierarchy. Being able to scribble down a 'sketch' of something that I didn't have the words to explain and being able to show that to Rudi as part of our active discussion also helped to communicate some of my experiences in a more interactive way.

In-person meetings are also much more sensitive to body language, facial expressions and other non-verbal forms of communication. It is no surprise to know that we all pick up on various signals – tense shoulders and twitching knee reflecting stress or anxiety, or open arms and a relaxed posture indicating confidence and happiness. However, it also allows us to adopt a 'persona'.

I had long been used to the confidence that came when I put on a business suit for government meetings or conferences. The clothing became like a 'suit of armour', and as the person wearing it, I felt competent and able to respond to whatever questions came my way. I was at times tempted to don my corporate suit to go to my rehab sessions, to put on that professional persona and hide behind a veneer of competency. However, I knew deep inside that this wasn't the right way to proceed. The only way forward was to try to search for a way of communicating the disturbing and distressing things I was now experiencing, and try to explain my difficulty in managing these.

Having time to 'prepare' was important to me in managing my rehab discussions. Since my brain injury, I found it very difficult to 'think on the hoof' as quickly and spontaneously as I always used to do, and I also struggled with thinking about what I wanted to say and simultaneously finding the right words and actually speaking. My conversations were often punctuated by repeated 'um's and ah's', along with, at times, an inability to progress with a sentence without repeating the same word or phrase. As someone who had previously been very articulate, this was quite distressing, but I found that if I had time on my own to slowly think through and write things down in advance, then I would be ok on the day. Arriving at the clinic, I would sit in the room, and unfold my piece of paper as a 'cue sheet' for discussion. Knowing that I had it written down reduced my anxiety and helped me feel a bit more in control of our discussions. I was always grateful that Rudi would start each session by asking 'what would you like to talk about today?' To begin with, this felt odd. I had assumed that, as the clinician, Rudi would take the lead and direct the conversation. However, in putting the decision back in my court, I was able to feel a degree of ownership and autonomy in what we talked about, and how much I revealed at any particular time, not moving beyond what I felt comfortable sharing.

In having cognitive difficulties, I initially felt particularly vulnerable in sharing what was going on in my head, and it would take a while to trust the clinician, seated beside me in the room, with some of the things that were going on in my head.

Trust is a strange process, and there has been much written in psychology about developing a 'therapeutic alliance' (eg, 'Building the bond: Predictors of the alliance in neurorehabilitation', Rowlands, Coetzer & Turnbull, 2020). Knowing the theory was one thing but actually trusting someone who, although a clinical professional, is to all intents and purposes a stranger, is a lot more challenging. It made a difference actually meeting Rudi in person. Even though he was the consummate professional in that he said very little, if anything, about himself, there was still a lot that instilled trust even in the early days. Meeting in person, he came across as confident but not overbearing or domineering, quiet but not silent, an extraordinarily good listener, and honest without being harsh or judgemental. These were many of the attributes that I both valued and appreciated, which also helped to build up a sense of trust. It also helped that he seemed to share my love of the mountains, and had heard of the music of Leonard Cohen – all of those little details that come up in rehab discussions. I had a great deal of respect for his ability to 'hold a reflective shield' up to me, so that he could engage in our discussions in a way which focused on my brain injury and the effect this had on the aspects of life that were important to me, without disrupting that with his own personal opinions or preferences.

Although that trust did not appear immediately, it did get more established in the first couple of months of my rehabilitation sessions at the Brain Injury Service. In those initial three to four months, I felt that I was gradually making progress in understanding more about my brain injury, what it meant, and the fact that – although I was never going to be able to go back to being the person I used to be – there was potential for improvement and an opportunity to explore returning to some of my pre-accident activities. At that point, this story would have probably continued along a similar trajectory as many others with a traumatic brain injury, albeit accepting that everyone's journey is individual and subject to challenges along the way. Although I had stopped work in January 2020 as I could no longer cope due to my brain injury, and I had withdrawn from most social engagement, I was hoping that my rehabilitation sessions with Rudi would slowly provide me with the knowledge and techniques I would need to try to return to some of these activities, or at least explore whether or not this was a viable option for me.

Then in February and March 2020, we were notified about a new virus, starting in China and rapidly spreading into other countries. My rehab journey then suddenly took on a whole new direction. Covid-19 presented significant changes and challenges to both people with a brain injury and to the whole of the NHS, including the clinicians at the North Wales Brain Injury Service. The world shut down and turned upside down for all of us.

The rest of this book explores the impact that had on rehabilitation from both perspectives – that of clinicians and that of people with a brain injury.

References

Elwick, H., Smith, L., Mhizha-Murira, J. R., Topcu, G., Leighton, P., Drummond, A., Evangelou, N., & das Nair, R. (2022). Cognitive assessment in multiple sclerosis clinical care: A qualitative evaluation of stakeholder perceptions and preferences. *Neuropsychological Rehabilitation*, *32*(7), 1456–1474. https://doi.org/10.1080/09602 011.2021.1899942

Hobden, G., Tang, E., & Demeyere, N. (2023). Cognitive assessment after stroke: A qualitative study of patients experiences. *BMJ Open*, *13*, e072501.

Maas, A. I. R., Menon, D. K., Manley, G. T., Abrams, M., Åkerlund, C., Andelic, N., Aries, M., Bashford, T., Bell, M. J., Bodien, Y. G., Brett, B. L., Büki, A., Chesnut, R. M., Citerio, G., Clark, D., Clasby, B., Cooper, D. J., Czeiter, E., Czosnyka, M., Dams-O'Connor, K., … InTBIR Participants and Investigators. (2022). Traumatic brain injury: Progress and challenges in prevention, clinical care, and research. *The Lancet. Neurology*, *21*(11), 1004–1060. https://doi.org/10.1016/S1474-4422(22)00309-X

National Neurosciences Advisory Group. (2023, May). *Optimal clinical pathway for adults: Traumatic brain injury.*

Rowlands, L., Coetzer, R., & Turnbull, O. H. (2020). Building the bond: Predictors of the alliance in neurorehabilitation. *NeuroRehabilitation*, *46*(3), 271–285. https://doi.org/10.3233/NRE-193005

Part 2

Covid-19

Chapter 3

All Change

The Pandemic Begins ...

Sue Williams and Rudi Coetzer

(i) Overview

In early 2020, the last thing most of us were expecting was the arrival of a pandemic that would rapidly spread across the world like a viral version of the charging horsemen of the apocalypse. The disturbing news of this new 'Corona Virus' added to the difficulties I was already having. Despite having recently started a process of rehabilitation with Rudi at the North Wales Brain Injury Service, this was still very early days and there was much about my brain injury that I didn't understand or knew how to manage. I was struggling with the increasingly overwhelming effects of my brain injury, including cognitive confusion and neurological fatigue. On top of which, a few months earlier, my much-loved disabled brother had died suddenly at the age of 47, devastating to all of us in our close-knit family, especially my mother, who had cared for him throughout his life. Loss and grief pushed me towards attempting my default coping mechanism of burying myself in work, trying to block out the emotions with demanding research and working longer hours. It didn't take long for this increased cognitive demand, combined with neurological fatigue, to exacerbate the effects of

DOI: 10.4324/9781003509134-6

my brain injury and push my fragile capability over the edge. I dropped out of work and struggled to see family or friends. I felt isolated, vulnerable, grief-stricken and guilty about not being there for my brother and above all, confused and scared by the increasingly disturbing effects of a brain which no longer functioned in a way I could understand or explain.

Into this complex mix came Covid-19 and the psychological, cognitive and practical challenges it presented to us all. In March 2020, life became very scary and challenging for everyone. The news had developed into a 'war footing' with national announcements from the Prime Minister. Society appeared at times to be disintegrating, with fights for food and empty supermarket shelves; friends and families said their goodbyes, hoping to meet up again; most workplaces shut down with little notice, as everyone was sent home. The NHS faced the most significant challenge, with staff staring into the face of a pandemic caused by a deadly new virus. The devastating images of sickness and death from across the world filled our screens, with some hospitals failing to cope with unsustainable levels of demand. All of this was now coming our way, and on March 23, the UK went into full lockdown, with the key message 'Stay Home, protect the NHS, Save Lives'. How did that core mantra affect both people like me, who needed on-going neurorehabilitation and clinicians like Rudi, who were essential to providing care during this exceptional time?

This chapter focuses on why and how the pandemic had such a profound effect on my neurorehabilitation in a diversity of ways, some more obvious than others. These included:

i. The delivery of NHS rehabilitation, in particular the risks and challenges of working within hospitals and that of home visits, along with the effects of changing from in-person to 'telehealth' methods.

ii. The mental health impact of increasing anxiety, fear and concern about the virus (both catching it and the risk of passing it on to others).

iii. Changes to critical support from family and friends, with strict limits on social contact and an increase in isolation.

iv. Practical changes to activities of daily living as we were all limited by what we could do, where we could go and the cognitive demands of managing these changes.

v. Impacts on the 'settings' for applying rehabilitation techniques, and changing opportunities for participation, with a sudden end to visiting the office or café, and a shift to outdoor-based activities.

The above areas presented significant challenges, not only for me as a patient but also for Rudi as my clinical neuropsychologist. In the immediate response to Covid-19, this was a journey that we had to walk together from both sides of the virtual desk, adjusting in real time to an ever-evolving situation without having previous experience of rehabilitation during a global pandemic with life-threatening consequences. This meant that neither of us was the 'expert', presenting an opportunity to dissolve some of the boundaries between clinical expertise and patient experience and gain greater insights from each other. As noted by Rudi in his review of the early impact of the pandemic on neurorehabilitation:

There has been a reduction in the gap between clinician and patient: we are in this together.

(Coetzer, 2020)

Coping with the pandemic was an exceptional challenge for all in the health sector, along with numerous other key workers. It was also difficult for people like myself with a brain injury, both in terms of how it affected us as individuals and also in our access to rehabilitation services. Exploring the impact of this through the lived experiences of both myself and Rudi offers an insight into how we navigated our way through this extraordinary time.

[Rudi]
Ours are two parallel, intermittently connected stories to tell a single, much broader story from the hundreds of thousands of stories of patients and clinicians who went through the pandemic. We saw the same images on the news, we read the same reports on what was happening, we drove past the same electronic road signs warning us in little orange dots to stay home, to keep safe. We also saw different things, some beautiful, some less so. More about these later. It is not a unique story per se, rather, a story of many different things. It's a story of the pandemic (of course), healthcare, society, communities and rehabilitation, amongst others, but ultimately it is a story of what it means to be human. Our fears, uncertainties, surprises and very occasionally the things that made us laugh or smile during the chaos of Covid-19 – all the emotions that make us human. And being human is what makes us all the same, but simultaneously unique, reflected here in our story about the pandemic.

(ii) Disconnecting: Saying Our Goodbyes

Even before the formal lockdown, we were all increasingly concerned about the risk of close contact with other people and the ease with which this new virus seemed to spread without necessarily having any visible symptoms or signs. In early March 2020, I met up for a couple of outdoor walks and picnics with a few close friends for a couple of outdoor walks and picnics, for what felt like possibly the last time. Although by then my circle of friends had been significantly diminished by the effects of my brain injury which had made socialising in normal places impossible due to the overwhelming pain in my head from multiple conversations and background noise, I was fortunate to have several very supportive friends who had always been on my 'brain injury journey' with me. This time, it wasn't just me that had to limit social contact, it was all of us.

Meeting outside for a walk, we tried to dissipate the fear with a bit of humour with a 'bum bump' at the start, on the basis that reversing with our bums meant that we were not going to accidentally breathe on each other! It was certainly more fun than the advocated 'elbow touch' of politicians. Despite the anxiety and the awkwardness of trying to stay far enough apart, there was so much value in the relative normality of seeing a friend in person and the benefits of human contact and support. My small circle of friends had become increasingly important to me over the previous year as I was already all too well versed in the negative impacts of social isolation, and I was dreading the effect of having my limited contact with a few friends reduced to

nothing. Waving goodbye, with the lockdown loom-
ing and incredible uncertainty about the virus and our
worries about whether we would even survive, we left
each other with a smile and the words 'see you on the
other side'.

[Rudi]
At a downtown local café and tap room for foodies, or
'pub-at-night', March 13, 2020. It is the normal after
work Friday informal socialising event with my uni-
versity academic colleagues at a popular local water-
ing hole and eatery. Beers from microbreweries is their
thing. Sometimes there is music too. Food, well yes, that
too, but not really during the evenings. That's a day-
time thing. Since 2015, for one day per week (Fridays), I
have been seconded from my full-time NHS role to teach
at our local university. My teaching is mainly in clinical
neuropsychology. With a tiny bit of research on the side-
line to make sure there's variety in the role. Enough of
academia, let's return to the pub.

It is not lost on me that it is Friday 13, but as a
clinician-scientist I am not superstitious. Evidence is
the primary currency, not opinions. However, there is
something about the date, and the news of a new virus
doing the rounds which necessitates our usual Friday
night outing to be enjoyed with something novel put in
place to protect us from this uninvited new viral visitor
to the world. It is called 'social distancing'. I have never
heard of the term before but now learn that it is a behav-
ioural approach to attempt to limit the spread of infec-
tions, going back to, for example, the flu pandemic of
1918 – 1919. For readers interested in learning more
about the 1918 – 1919 pandemic, I highly recommend
Catharine Arnold's book, Pandemic 1918.

Like many before me, and now, I had failed to learn from history. At this point, I viewed the new virus as something that 'will go away within the next few weeks', nothing to worry about. At most, a disrupting annoyance. It reminded me a bit of the disruption to travel caused by the 2010 volcanic ash cloud. The next day, my friend and I were flying to South Africa via Germany for a holiday we had been looking forward to throughout the unrelenting, bleak British winter. By the time we come back, surely all this business of a virus will be over and already forgotten, and in a month we'll all be back in the pub after work. Plus, the clocks would have changed by then, and it would be much lighter. It was probably one of my worst predictions. Ever.

Little did I know that Friday March 13, 2020 was to be the last after work socialisation with my academic colleagues for a very long time. The next time I was to see them was many months later, in a different world. Virtually, just digital avatars of the people I was with every Friday for the past five years. I could see them, but I could not reach out and touch them. Everything was visual, with an auditory top-up. Wow, look at their hair! It has grown tremendously since Friday March 13, 2020! Ah, there's one of their kids in the background. And they have a stripey cat, I didn't know that. Why are they looking at me blankly now? Oh no! I have yet again forgotten to unmute myself. Here in the wards, I've fallen so far behind with my tech skills...

For now, though, this weekend of March 13 – 15, 2020, the world was still analogue and tangible. Besides Manchester Airport being unexpectedly very quiet and the fact that there was lots of parking, the actual flight to South Africa on Saturday went fine, arriving at Oliver Tambo airport on the Sunday morning. However, when after a long period of nothing happening after landing, the South African National Defence Force boarded the plane, I had an overwhelming sense that maybe something was not quite right. Maybe Manchester Airport was quiet for a reason yesterday? Here at Oliver Tambo Airport now, every passenger had to have their temperature taken before anyone would be allowed to disembark.

Row after row, thermometer inserted into the ears of all passengers, the figures in camouflage systematically went about their task of checking for anyone who had a fever. You could faintly hear the beeps when they were taking temperatures in your row. Their faces gave nothing away. After some delay, the announcement came that everybody could disembark. Stepping off the plane, the light outside was intense and blue after being confined to a noisy metal tube with artificial lighting for too many hours. It was nice to be back in the sun of Africa and breathe in the warm fresh air. Little did I know that soon breathing in fresh air for many would soon take on a new meaning. Fresh air and to be able to breathe freely, was soon to become something very precious, something to be grateful for, something to be savoured and a lack of this, for many, was a nightmare.

(iii) Lockdown March 23, 2020

Sue's Journal March 23, 2020

4am … the night-time horrors have left me wide awake again. I hate these nightmares – the blood, the gore, the torture … the inability to act

or intervene ... the sense of being utterly powerless to stop the horror of what is happening. I don't
understand why I get these horrific dreams, they
are worse now than they were after my accident.
I guess I'll just have to accept them as part of the
daily disrupted sleep that comes with my damaged
brain. At least I no longer need an alarm clock when
I wake up at 3 or 4am every day.

I'm tired, so very, very tired, I always am nowadays. My brain can't manage to keep up with
doing even the simplest of 'everyday' things. Why
is the world so busy all the time? Even in these
strange and increasingly silent days. Everything
is changing; it's so scary. The last few days feel
like society is breaking down; two men were fighting in the supermarket over food yesterday. I need
a regular routine, things in the same place in the
shops. I don't know how I'm going to manage as
everything changes.

As usual, the nightmares sent my adrenalin pump-
ing, typical 'fight or flight'. It drove me out of bed
despite the darkness and the early hour. I had to get
out to escape from what was going on in my head.

So I slipped like a silent wraith out of the house
into the cool darkness before dawn. Despite the
lack of light, I felt safe out there at that time. There
was no-one else about, my ears strained to detect
the slightest of sounds, but the world still sleeps.
The threat of this new virus that stalks the land is
muted when there is no-one around, but I still walk
down the white line in the centre of the road. The
sensation that 'something' is out there to get me is

too strong, and I try to avoid the driveway entrances and garden hedges that line the road. Memories of my accident and that unseen car suddenly emerging from a side turning seem to be permanently stuck in my mind. 'Red' 'Blood' 'Pain' repeat like a mantra in my brain.

This morning the sea was calling, providing a sense of solace in the sound of the waves. The beach was empty at dawn, this is the safest place to be. The ebbing tide has washed the sand clean, a natural blank canvas. The lack of even a single footprint provides clear, incontrovertible evidence of the absence of any threat; no-one else has been this way today. As I walked across the shifting sands towards the sea, there was nothing to disrupt my gaze. There is little sensory stimulation to tax my struggling brain; it feels like a brief respite from a head full of pain.

Ever since my accident, I have found relief in the silence of empty landscapes. My injured brain can no longer cope with man made sounds, the hectic movement of people, or the visual complexity of human interventions in the surrounding land. Even more so now when we have to avoid people to stay safe and save lives.

Out here I feel safe again – the adrenalin that has got me here subsides, replaced by a sense of serenity and calm as my breathing found a shared natural harmony with the ebb and flow of the tide. All too soon, I had to go home and hide; we are not allowed out after today so I won't be safe outside again.

[Rudi]

Inside the belly of T5, Heathrow Airport, London, UK, March 21, 2020. T5 is deserted. I've never seen it like this. All the shops are closed. There are hardly any people about. Disbelieving, I take a couple of photos to remind myself that 'this is real, I am not imagining what I am seeing.' What a relief to be back in the UK, after being stuck in Africa for a week. A few hours after arriving there for a long-awaited three-week holiday and clearing the on-plane temperature checking, in response to Covid-19, the South African borders were closed, social control implemented, and almost all return flights out of the country suspended. During that week of overwhelming uncertainty, I reminded myself (many times!), that 'every problem has a solution', and that is how, through staying calm and the immeasurable kindness of people I knew from a past life and who 'took us in', that I now found myself inside an eerily quiet T5. It all feels like a dream, but one where you wake up and the bad dream you were having really is what is happening in the awake world. A snooze on the connecting flight doesn't help dispel the dream, I'm awakened by someone coughing, something with new meaning since a week ago.

Sunday, March 22, 2020
Despite a sleep of oblivion after a long-haul flight, gradually during the day the realisation that this is bad – Covid-19 is more than real and won't blow over in a few weeks – starts to sink into my long-haul befuddled brain. The signs within society and the media are that it is unlike anything else we've seen in recent memory.

They are right. Covid-19, and how to manage it, was 'not on the curriculum' in our clinical training. We fear the things we don't know anything about, leaving vast tracts of cognitive space for us to ruminate, weigh up, assume and conclude the inevitably bleak insights that occur in a vacuum of knowledge. But I already suspect that besides the likely very high physical mortality, there is almost certainly going to be profound mental health consequences too, for everyone.

In a feeble attempt to try and reduce that risk for myself, I make a commitment to exercise outside in fresh air every day and stay fit until the pandemic is over. Maybe it wasn't the classic defining and committing to a goal. Perhaps it was more of a 'doing nothing is even worse than at least trying something'. The reason being that it was now clearly time to return to work, the NHS, and I needed to be well enough to be able to make my small contribution to patient care during the pandemic. A hike out to the lowest mountain in England and Wales, Tal y Fan on Sunday March 22, 2020 was the beginning of that journey. There are many many photographs that I took during these days outside in nature. Little did I know whilst dragging a tired body over soggy moorland towards tiny Tal y Fan, that the mountains the next 18 months of Covid-19 would bring to all of us to climb over, would be huge, and that everything as we knew it in the hospital and society was going to change. On March 9, 2025 I took what is probably my last 'pandemic photograph'. It was the UK Covid-19 Day of Reflection, and I had walked back to Tal y Fan, where I took a photo of the trigpoint under a beautiful blue sky.

Everything changed as soon as lockdown began in the UK. The Prime Minister's national television announcement on March 23, 2020 was stark in its reference to this 'invisible killer' and the real risk of the NHS becoming overrun and unable to cope with the potentially huge number of people becoming seriously ill and dying from the virus. At that point, the only option available was to prevent as much contact between people as possible to try to stop transmission.

The strict instructions were essential and clear (PM Speech March 23, 2020):

People will only be allowed to leave their home for the following very limited purposes:

- Shopping for basic necessities, as infrequently as possible;
- One form of exercise a day – for example a run, walk, or cycle – alone or with members of your household;
- Any medical need, to provide care or to help a vulnerable person; and
- Travelling to and from work, but only where this is absolutely necessary and cannot be done from home.

That's all – these are the only reasons you should leave your home.

This changed everything, for everyone. It created a society where the majority were limited to life within their own houses except for 'daily exercise'. However, essential services were still required, especially hospitals, which were critical for treating both Covid-19 patients and others with serious unavoidable illness and injuries, leading to a new group – 'Key Workers' – who became even more valued and appreciated by all in our communities.

[Rudi]
Being identified as a key worker meant I could come and go, a passport of sorts, to the world outside home. It was not a feeling of freedom though. No, the sense of being restricted was overwhelming. The only daily drive, on deserted roads, was to a hospital, another NHS clinical setting, or doing a home visit in the community. And then back home at the end of the day. No variation in how you dress – the same colour (blue – although this did change later, see below) of scrubs plus personal protective equipment (PPE, i.e., in my case, masks, gloves, plastic protection over scrubs, sometimes a visor, and so forth) every day. My world lost its colour, and the groove I fell into with time, became very deep. Hospital coffee every day, no quick nipping out to a nearby coffee shop. After work, a walk later in the evening, often in the dark, when it was quiet. Other than my friend at home, no other social contact. Her life was even more isolated. Staying at home, working remotely, staring at a screen until her eyes saw double, no, triple, every day. With the added factor of a key worker who had potentially been exposed to Covid-19 every day, arriving home in the evening.

Simple things like shopping became complicated. Want to bake a bread? Think again. People have been stockpiling flour and yeast. Your car needs a service? You better start hoping that the oil will not turn even blacker and the spark plugs keep firing for a little while longer. And sometimes, though not often, complicated things became simple... For example, a local pizzeria where the owner simply spray-painted a carefully measured semi-circular red line at the entrance to the place – stand behind the line and shout what you'd like to order for your supper! Or parking, yes parking at the hospital became simple. Or later on, scrubs. After one of my colleagues said to me, winking, when I arrived back at our unit, 'what's up with the blue scrubbies Roots, what if they ask you to catch a baby in the corridor', it was a simple matter of deciding a colour, confirm the embroidery (for identification of profession) and order them. For the record, it was purple I chose. Perhaps I had a slight fever when I chose my colour! But at least it would be difficult to lose me in a sea of blue. And maybe subconsciously purple is my colour...

(iv) Silence Falls: An Oasis for my Brain

Lockdown: For the first time ever, the country fell silent and a deep hush settled across the land like a blanket of heavy snow. It felt like everything had stopped: no cars, no voices, no movement outside. It was an incredibly surreal experience, as if everyone in the country had just disappeared.

The last thing I expected at the start of lockdown was an overwhelming sense of cognitive relief. Surely nothing good could possibly come out of something so awful as locking away everyone in their own homes? Despite my fear and anxiety about the virus, along with concern for my family and friends, the silence of lockdown simultaneously provided a sudden respite from the clamour of everyday life and the overwhelming impact this usually had on my brain.

Sue's Journal March 26, 2020

It's quiet, so quiet out there today. I woke up and opened the window this morning and the only thing I could hear was the sound of the birds. It is so beautifully tranquil. Nothing moving, no-one rushing around, no cars revving as everyone goes to work. I know I shouldn't think this, given how awful everything is with the virus and how many people are suffering, but it feels so good for my brain. It's quiet and peaceful for the first time. My headache has stopped, and it feels like a huge strain has left my mind. The continuous effort has gone and I can rest my brain now. I don't have to try to keep up with everything and I don't feel like I'm always failing and trailing behind. I'm scared of the virus too, like everyone else, but this silence just feels like an oasis for my brain.

I had spent the last 18 months since my accident wishing the world would be quiet, just for a while, so my brain could have a rest from always trying to process and pay attention to everything. Now it had, and although I was scared and isolated like everyone else due to this horrific new virus, I was at the same time grateful for the respite it provided to my overloaded brain. I kept this sudden revelation hidden as it felt so wrong to feel that there was anything positive about the terrible situation we had all been forced into, but at the same time I could not deny the beneficial impact that the silence had on my brain.

[Rudi]
Silence is like a special medicine for an overwhelmed brain. People who have sustained a traumatic brain injury often describe an overwhelming sense of relief when they suddenly find themselves in a quiet environment or situation that is not perceptually overwhelming. Some of the examples of this dramatic transition from overstimulation to peace that I have heard described to me as a clinician over the years include walking on a beach at night, doing a solo hike in the mountains, swimming (being underwater), running, or the first time using noise-cancelling headphones. On the other hand, some of the worst environments concerning over-stimulation for someone with processing difficulties or noise sensitivity, I have been told about by patients, are supermarkets (consistently), train stations and airports, among others.

Being in these noisy, busy environments can have a range of profound emotional responses – for example, an overwhelming sense of panic, wanting to immediately leave or flee, a sense of 'having lost their mind', or becoming agitated. I've even been told (more than once) that in desperation, shopping had to be left in the trolley to flee what must have felt like such a hostile environment to the person. A recent paper by Wilson et al. (2021) highlights the important relationship between impaired processing and everyday functioning for people who have sustained a traumatic brain injury. It makes complete sense that Sue found some respite when the world went quiet during the start of the pandemic. Below, Sue provides a unique 'insider's account' that clinical textbooks simply cannot capture, through a more detailed phenomenological account of what difficulties with processing actually feels like to her, as well reflecting as an academic on her experiences.

My initial neuropsychological test results had shown that the damage to my brain meant that I now had a very slow 'processing speed', difficulties with managing attention, along with executive dysfunction. 'Why is the world so noisy and busy?' used to be my constant refrain, as I struggled to cope and became overwhelmed over and over again. Yet it wasn't that the world had suddenly become more hectic since my accident, it was because my brain could no longer keep up with everything, from the smallest of sounds, to movement, lights, emails and innumerable daily conversations. Nor could my brain manage to pay attention to the 'right' things and instead it would try to give equal attention to every competing aspect of sound, light, conversation and movement around me. It is no wonder that it didn't take much for everyday life to completely overwhelm me. Every second of every day, my brain strained to process the myriad of stimuli that came hurtling my way. Inevitably, it would lead to a cognitive car crash in my brain, and I would often completely shut down – physically, mentally and emotionally – even in the middle of the day.

It has taken me a long time to understand the reasons for the difficulties I have in noisy and busy situations. I used to only think 'Pay Attention' applied only to errant pupils in a schoolroom! I certainly never realised that 'attention' was a complex cognitive function that applies to everything we experience in normal life. Attention is also the essential foundation for other cognitive activities, such as remembering things, communicating, learning, processing information, decision making and completing tasks. In other words, problems with attention cause significant difficulties with many other cognitive processes, and the impact of attention impairments often causes overwhelm, anxiety and even 'brain freeze' – a form of cognitive self-protection that shuts everything down, even the ability to move or speak. I frequently experience this, and it is something which causes me great distress and social embarrassment if it occurs in front of other people and results in overwhelming neurological fatigue, often lasting for days.

I have difficulties with the following 'types of attention' (I never realised this was more than one type of process, but have learnt that attention has several components):

- Selective Attention: the ability to select and respond to the right stimuli whilst simultaneously filtering out other competing unimportant stimuli.
- Sustained Attention: maintaining concentration on a particular task (such as reading a book), without getting distracted by internal or external things.
- Alternating Attention: the ability to switch between tasks, stopping one activity to do something else, and then successfully returning to the original task.
- Divided Attention: the ability to pay attention to doing more than one thing at once, for example, walking and navigating a route, or talking to a passenger whilst driving.

The silence of the Covid-19 lockdown particularly helped with my extreme difficulties with 'Selective Attention'. I have great difficulty in selectively focusing on specific stimuli (ie the person I am talking to or the book I am reading), whilst simultaneously filtering out all other stimuli (for example, other conversations, cars passing, people moving around, etc). It is therefore clear why the almost total cessation of background noise, movement and other 'normal' everyday activities that happened during the initial lockdown, had such a beneficial effect on my brain.

Many of us with a brain injury struggle with attention and have difficulties with its various forms. A fellow brain injury survivor, Aurora Lassaletta, describes in detail the challenges she has with selective attention and the issues this presents for managing everyday life in her excellent book on the lived experience of having an 'Invisible Brain Injury' (Lassaletta, 2020). Like myself, this causes immense difficulties with undertaking practical activities in certain situations, for example, needing complete silence from others whilst trying to read or drive a car.

I soon learnt with my brain injury that it is very difficult to expect or require the person you are with, or even the rest of the population, to 'please be quiet'. My partner and close friends have been incredibly supportive of my difficulties and will do their best to remain silent when they know I am struggling, but even for them, this can be a 'big ask' at times, especially when even the sound of someone breathing next to me can be overwhelming at times. So my usual approach is to withdraw from most situations which are even slightly noisy or busy, or sadly at times, from being with anyone at all, which frequently leaves me socially isolated.

Lassaletta (2020) refers to the cognitive overload that comes from being exposed to too many auditory, visual, cognitive and emotional stimuli as 'saturation'. Her co-author, neuropsychologist Amor Bize, notes:

> People with brain injury often avoid family dinners, weekend trips to shopping centres and, in general, any situation that means they will be bombarded by visual and / or auditory stimuli. The capacity we have to differentiate important information from unimportant information and to allocate processing resources only to the former, is often lost, which means that people "have to" pay attention to each and every one of the stimuli they receive, and this is why the processing system collapses in these situations.
>
> (Bize in Lassaletta, 2020)

The Covid-19 lockdown managed to achieve something that in normal circumstances would have been impossible, and it is therefore not surprising that my brain found solace in the silence of this first lockdown. Suddenly, instead of having to 'self-isolate' myself from exposure to most social situations and other people, the country as a whole withdrew into their own homes. Cafés and shops shut down, workplaces and schools were closed, roads and playgrounds were empty. The country stood still and silent. Consequently, the total level of background stimulus (noise, movement, visual information etc) became completely muted, and silence descended across the land. Instead of me having to withdraw from the world, the world shut down around me, and for once, I felt the peace that I craved so much to rest my brain.

[Rudi] April 21, 2020
The world has gone astonishingly quiet. There is an
absence of movement and sound. It is so quiet; you
can hear your own thoughts. The quietness makes all
visual stimuli feel much more intense, looking at things
now seems to require more processing than before. It
feels like it takes more time to 'see' things properly.
I took three photographs today of the motorway run-
ning through North Wales. There is no traffic. In both
directions. I wonder which direction the pandemic will
go? Another photograph I took on the same day shows
a public bin, taped closed with red and white ribbon,
incongruously on a deserted, sunny beach. A bright yel-
low Council road sign says in stern black letters that the
centre is closed, we should go home, and save lives. For
a moment, I wonder where my home now really is. I'm
not sure if it is at home anymore.

It was not just the silence that made the difference, but
many things also seemed to slow down. A lot of people
took a deep breath and paused as we tried to adjust to
this sudden change. As someone whose brain injury had
left them with a significantly 'slow speed of processing',
this was also a blessing in disguise. Before the Covid-19
lockdown, I had been 'out of step' with everyone else
who could continue with life at their normal pace. With
lockdown, the monumental cognitive effort of trying to
process everything around me and trying to keep up with
everyone temporarily stopped. It was such a relief and
the respite that this gave to my brain came at such a critical time. The previous 18 months of trying to recover,
attempting to 'fit in', and to go back to my normal life
had taken so much out of me. I had not yet learned that

my brain needed extra time and rest throughout the day, and I would in the future need to develop strategies to manage the daily bombardment that everyday life would send my way.

The timing of this silence and societal slowdown was important in my rehab journey. For over a year, I had been overloading my brain on a daily basis, lacking the knowledge and skills required to provide the required respite for my brain. Unlike a broken leg, where a plaster cast can hold the bone immobile whilst it repairs itself, I had no idea how to 'rest' my brain. The consequence of that was repeated periods of neurological 'boom' and 'bust', until it reached the stage where 'bust' became an almost permanent situation. Nowadays, I have a range of strategies that I use on a daily basis, from changing my home environment to remove all unnecessary auditory stimuli (there are no ticking clocks or radios in my house), to the use of ear defenders and black out curtains, along with mindfulness techniques. But back in early 2020, I tried to 'rest' by watching TV, reading a book, or lying in bed staring at the ceiling whilst trying my best 'not to think'. Unsurprisingly, none of these approaches worked.

So in many ways, the lockdown provided me with critical respite and an opportunity to rest my brain from over-stimulation, to slowly recover some capacity and to reduce my neurological fatigue at a time when I needed it most. If the lockdown had happened now, five years after my accident, when I have learnt various strategies to self-manage some my difficulties with selective attention and processing, then I do not think the societal silence would have had such an impact on providing a rest for my brain, although I still seek out quiet places today.

[Rudi] May 22, 2020
A photograph I took today of a couple of swings tied
together in the middle to prevent children from playing
there confirms the fact that we are still in lockdown. The
beautifully symmetrical blue and red metal frame stands
motionless in the bright Spring sunshine. The little play-
ing park by the sea is quiet. I become aware my pho-
tographs are quiet too. There's either no people in the
photographs, or just the one, same person every time.
While my life inside the hospital is full of sound and
movement every day, life outside is quiet and isolated.
I find this peaceful, and a relief every day after work.
The sound of the waves has never before sounded so
reassuring.

I was not alone in finding a sense of relief in this 'slowing down' of society. Whilst many people embraced the
opportunity to live a slightly less hectic life, it was particularly significant for those of us who experience high
levels of cognitive and sensory overload, and therefore
struggle to manage everyday demands, such as people
with a brain injury, autism or dementia.

A qualitative study of the experience of partners of
people with an acquired brain injury (ABI) during the
first Covid-19 lockdown highlighted the importance
and benefit of 'slowing down' for both themselves [the
partner] and the person with an ABI:

> Slowing down the pace of life was not only of benefit
> to the participant, but they observed benefits in their
> loved one, identifying that this was now important
> for the long term (not just the lock down period). "It
> just meant everything slowed down so it was a calmer

pace of life, it was an easier pace of life ... and I think that probably helped with [their] recovery as well.

(Beal et al., 2023)

However, there appears to be little research that has explored the impact of the reduction in external stimuli on people with a brain injury during the pandemic. In addition to the potential benefits, depending on how important this aspect is the person with a brain injury, there is also limited discussion on the effect this had on the longer-term progression of rehabilitation.

Whilst I found immense relief in silence and the societal slowdown, I had little idea how long this would go on for in these first few months of the pandemic. Nor was I aware of the risk that this would develop into an ongoing 'avoidance behaviour' with longer-term consequences for hypersensitivity. These were challenges that would only become apparent in the future. In the present, just like everyone else, I was just focused on trying to cope with the changing life that managing the virus had brought to us all.

(v) Welcome to my World!

In the early days of the pandemic, one of the key strategies to try to reduce transmission of the virus was to significantly restrict in-person interactions. We were all limited to only having contact with the people within our own household, which was very hard for people living alone. The first lockdown introduced a whole new terminology, and we all became used to talking about 'social distancing' and 'self-isolation'. But for someone like me, these lockdown restrictions were already all too familiar because of the difficulties I had in social situations due to my brain injury.

> Sue's Journal April 3, 2020
> Welcome to my World! I can't really say this to anyone, and I wouldn't want to wish it on my worst enemy, but this 'social isolation' isn't new to me. My brain injury means I've not been able to get together with many people for a long time now. I'm OK if it's just one or two people at a time, but any more than that fries my brain. So I haven't been going to things with groups of friends for ages, and I've really missed that. I doubt anyone really noticed, as it didn't particularly affect them. I guess, if nothing else, I've got some experience of not seeing people in person very much anymore. At least now we are all in the same boat, and I'm not always on my own on the outside looking in.

As a clinician, Rudi's world was very different to mine. He faced the challenge of immediately changing practices in the North Wales Brain Injury Service, from the cessation of in-clinic appointments to arranging telephone check-ins. In contrast to me, when it came to clinical home visits, he was the person who was 'on the outside and coming in'. These home visits to people with a brain injury were essential in some cases and presented significant concerns for all, especially in the early days of lockdown. His journal entries below show the range of issues that presented in his world of change.

[Rudi] March 31, 2020
I did a home visit today, of someone whom I had seen for
long-term follow-up. There was no choice in the matter
to do a home visit when considering the clinical risks
related to their brain injury. It would be irresponsible,
and lacking in any humanity, to not see them to find out
how they are during these extraordinary times, as well
as do a clinical review. Whilst putting on my personal
protective equipment (PPE) outside of my car, I noticed
out of the corner of my eye that they are watching me
very intently from inside their house as I get ready.
Inside, I feel like the guest who misread the dress code
on an invite to a wedding. It's like I am wearing a 10mm
neoprene wetsuit whereas I should have gone down
the Hugo Boss route instead. Ugly, warm, noisy and
uncomfortable.

Every time I move, the rustle of plastic reminds me
that I am over (no, under?) dressed for this special-
but-routine situation. When I leave, I have a sense of
unease – do we know exactly how contagious this virus
is? Were they protected from me, and I from them?
Looking at the crumpled up little heap of used Personal
Protective Equipment (PPE) in the trunk of my car as
I get rid of my forced choice outfit for the visit, I wonder
if PPE is really such a robust barrier? The grey colour
and rough texture of the carpet on the floor of the boot
of my car is clearly visible through the green plastic of
the now extensively creased and discarded apron. The
blue gloves put up a slightly better defence against the
reality check of translucence, whilst the light blue mask
just slightly smirks back at me, expressionless, making
no promises. Oh well, there is always alcohol to save

me! I lavishly apply the hand gel to clean my hands but then have to wait for my slippery hands to dry before I can safely drive.

April 6, 2020
A day spent at the unit figuring out how we will continue to provide clinical input, through a combination of remote and direct contact with those in our care. All unit-based appointments have been cancelled. We will, for now, as a default approach 'reach out, or remote out'. Reaching out will be very important. The pandemic is depriving people of all human contact and increasingly isolating them. There is something about the presence of another soul. Added to that, it's not exactly easy to remotely optimally perform some (not all) of the neuropsychological assessments and interventions we do.

April 9, 2020
A home visit to see a new referral. It's not easy to do an initial clinical assessment through the physical and psychological barrier that is PPE. I wish I could have done a better assessment and feel frustrated trying to do that with 'my hands tied behind my back'. Leaving, as we say goodbye at the front door, I am humbled by the gratitude they express that someone from the hospital has managed to come out, to see them in person. They've not seen a soul since the start of Lockdown.

April 15, 2020
I find out how exhausting and draining telephone consultations are. On the other side of the telephone, voices palpable with anxiety about the pandemic, panic about when in-person outpatient appointments will come

*back, and already the early signs of loneliness and iso-
lation for some. As a clinician, it is difficult to form an
accurate picture of how someone is doing when you
have no visual cues. Voices are electronically distorted,
and sometimes the signal breaks up, or there is background noise. And what to make of long silences? There
is also the uncomfortable feeling that someone at the
end of the telephone conversation is left uncontained,
often alone, at home, after discussing things that were
anxiety provoking or upsetting for them.*

The previous 18 months before the Covid-19 Lockdown
had been increasingly upsetting as I had tried over and
over again to fit in with groups of friends or go to various
work conferences and meetings. The pain in my head
and the cognitive overload from trying to cope with all
the background noise and conversations meant that I
had no choice but to withdraw from meeting people. If
I tried, I was left exhausted and overcome with neurological fatigue for days or even weeks at a time. No-one
wants to be isolated, to not be able to join in, and it felt
extremely distressing to have to say no to meeting up
with many of my friends. I missed out on so much that
I had previously enjoyed and felt disconnected from the
shared experience the everyday life of weekends away,
going to the café or restaurant, and the buzz of ideas at
work meetings and international conferences.

At the same time, I appreciated how fortunate I was to
have a supportive partner, family, and some very close
friends. I had already learnt early on that my brain injury
meant that I could only cope with meeting only one or
two people at a time, ideally somewhere quiet with no
background noise. I will remain forever grateful to those

people in my life who changed some parts of their social life too in order to meet up with me and accommodate my different needs. They accepted that I could no longer do simple things, like go to the café with them for a coffee, and that all too often my neurological fatigue made me unreliable and frequently too tired to meet up with them as planned. However, although I appreciated the efforts of this small number of key friends, I still missed out on so much, and frequently felt left out and excluded from so many activities and events.

Social isolation is recognised as a significant issue for many people with a brain injury, especially in relation to managing this chronic condition over the longer-term as friendships end, social networks reduce, and new contacts become harder to initiate, develop and maintain (Salas et al., 2016). Numerous personal accounts of brain injury survivors have emphasised the immediate impact that their brain injury has on limiting their social life, and the subsequent increase in social isolation.

[Rudi]
Social isolation among people with traumatic brain injury (TBI) was indeed one of the most important adverse consequences of the pandemic. Morrow et al. (2021) reported findings from their study in the United States which showed that a third of the population found that having had a traumatic brain injury made coping with the pandemic more challenging; the main contributors being mental health difficulties and social isolation. In many cases, patients' rehabilitation slowed down or stagnated. However, some people did report that the simplification or slowing down of life in general did help them, especially with regards to not being able

to visit or travel to very busy, noisy environments they would have been exposed to as part of their daily routines pre-pandemic. For these people, lockdown and the general slowing in pace of everyday life did bring some welcome respite from their sensitivity to cognitive and perceptual overload.

Before the Covid-19 lockdown, I felt like I was living in an impenetrable glass box. I could see out at everyone getting together, laughing, talking and having fun. They could look over and see me standing there and would beckon to encourage me to come and join them. But I couldn't, the effect of my brain injury – the pain, confusion and overload – acted as a barrier. I was trapped inside an invisible glass box, able to see out but unable to join in. But to everyone else, I still looked the same, like the 'old me', and they often didn't realise, or couldn't understand, why I could not come along or join them in the same way.

So when the Covid-19 lockdown started I was unfortunately already experienced in a life of 'social distancing' and 'isolation'. Whilst I had no wish to welcome anyone else into 'my world' of limited social interaction, the lockdown restrictions meant that now we all faced a shared challenge of coping without seeing other people in person. Instead of feeling like the 'odd one out', the person who saw everyone else going out and having fun whilst knowing that I couldn't join in, suddenly I felt part of the community again. We were all now concerned about social isolation, especially its impact on mental health and well-being, and were all worried about our friends and family, especially anyone we knew who was living on their own during the time when we were only allowed to mix with our own 'household'.

Communities, friends and strangers all came together during this crisis and showed extraordinary levels of caring and initiative, doing everything they could to stay connected and support each other. Across my diverse social network, many of whom I had known for years prior to my brain injury, we reached out to each other in a show of solidarity. As soon as lockdown began, my phone started pinging with messages of support and suggestions for online activities.

I am fortunate that, despite my cognitive difficulties, I was still quite capable of using technology and could access many online platforms such as zoom and teams. To my surprise, I found that I could now join in the same as everyone else, I was part of a wider social life again, albeit online, thanks to the innovative and pro-active activities of several friends. I 'went' to the movies with a regular online film night and a follow-on group zoom chat as we all dialled in at the same time to talk about the film we had just watched 'together but apart' in our own homes. Best of all was being asked if I wanted to join some kind of 'Dance Party'! I must admit my first inclination was to say no, I wasn't convinced by the idea of logging on to my laptop with a bunch of other people with a nominated 'DJ' who would play a few songs whilst we danced away at home. But I had missed the laughter of a party, and the fun of dancing, so I thought I'd give it a go. After all, I could always just join once, say I'd tried it, and then never go again. However, without doubt it became one of my favourite 'lockdown' activities, the perfect mix of chatting, happy music and physical movement. It is remarkable that

'Dance Party' has continued after lockdown, and five years later I still join in as it is the only way with a brain injury that I can go dancing with my friends.

So in some ways, the Covid-19 lockdown opened the social door again for me. I was on a level playing field with everyone else; we all faced the same challenge of not being able to see people in person and having to only connect online. For the first time in 18 months, I was now able to say 'yes' to various social invites, and to make an active contribution to organising activities myself. It felt so good to be part of things again, albeit in the strange, lockdown, online way.

[Rudi] May 24, 2020, 19:22
The promenade by the beach is quiet. The photograph I have just taken is of a beautifully painted stone. One of many left by people to connect to each other and say thank you to the NHS and other key workers. Blue, with a bright green grass blade and some delicate purple, pink and yellow dots to complement the main colours. Blue and green are colours I see every day. A lot. The stone is lying in the grass; the live grass almost seamlessly transitioning into the dead (paint) grass on the stone. The border between real and virtual grass is thin. The message painted on the stone is simple: 'Reset 2020'. I have failed to reset to the digital, virtual age. It is complicated to bring laptops into the wards, but not impossible. No, the failure is mine. I've, over the past couple of months, not stayed up-to-date with the new tech platforms. I don't really know how to use Teams, Zoom, or all the other variants available to make virtual contact with other people. I'm immersed in a world of three-dimensional people and analogue objects. My failure is

*that I am emotionally too drained to try and learn any-
thing new in the world of tech. My excuse is that I now
work in a world where very unwell, and lonely, people
without any social contact seem to crave the presence of
another, someone being there, sometimes asking (sometimes not) if they can touch my blue plastic hand. Not
answering that call feels very wrong.*

In addition to being able to join in as much as was possible in the limited online Covid-19 activities that had
sprung up during the pandemic, it meant a lot to me to
see the significant increase in awareness of the mental
health impacts of social isolation. Across society there
was a shared concern for others, about how they might
be coping with the isolation of lockdown, and how that
could lead to depression or anxiety. I really appreciated
this increased awareness and empathy. Although it was
primarily being driven by the constraints imposed to
manage the transmission of the virus, I benefited significantly as it helped address some of my isolation due
to my brain injury.

I am aware that I was fortunate enough to have a
range of factors in my favour that meant that, initially,
the Covid-19 lockdown left me feeling in some ways
included rather than excluded. In particular, I had the
capability to engage with online technology, had a
number of supportive friends, and was part of a wide
social network that had been established prior to my
accident. Many other people with a brain injury were
not so fortunate, and for them, the Covid-19 lockdown
left them even more isolated.

Despite the benefits of being able to join in online, I found that I deeply missed the personal contact with my close friends. There was a contrast between the relative expansion of my 'light touch' social network during the lockdown, and the reduction in my 'in-depth' friendship connections. The impact of this on perceived loneliness has been explored in discussions about the 'quantity' of social contact (for example, the size of a social network) and the 'quality' of that contact (loneliness as a subjective assessment).

The terms loneliness and social isolation have been often used interchangeably. However, they should be considered as two distinct concepts. Social isolation refers to a decreased quantity of social relations with other people (Zavaleta et al., 2014). Studies often conceptualize the quantity of social contact as the structural characteristics of a social network (size, composition, frequency and length of contact). In contrast, the quality of social contact has been defined as the individual's subjective assessment of how satisfied they are with their social relationships. Importantly, the qualitative interpretation that your social needs are not being met is the hallmark of loneliness. Moreover, several studies have shown that quantitative and qualitative components of social relationships are dissociable (Salas et al., 2021; Byrne et al., 2022). For example, a person may have a small social network but experience it as supportive, or have a large social network and feel lonely.

(Byrne et al., 2022)

The effects of my reduced in-depth and in-person social contact really began to bite as the pandemic progressed. However, in the early days, the expansion of my online social network and the benefits of being able to join in, along with the shared understanding and empathy of the impact of isolation and the ability to stay connected remotely whilst also being physically apart, helped me to overcome some of my pre-pandemic feelings of social isolation and exclusion that had been caused by the cognitive limitations of my brain injury.

[Rudi]
A bit of a loner, outside of work I've mostly kept to myself, preferring solitary activities. Before the pandemic my social connectedness was mainly through my colleagues at the community Brain Injury Service where I was based. During my secondment, I made several new work colleague-friends. These were the new colleagues I was working with. In particular, there was one ward where I spent a lot of time being involved in the care of inpatients who had sustained a brain injury (mostly Stroke) and who, despite the pandemic, still needed rehabilitation. Instead of individual offices, there was only one space available for all of us – the physiotherapy gym – which was where we spent our time together when not seeing patients by the bedside on the ward. 'The ward', with its separate bays, was in fact right outside the door of the gym. Step outside, turn right, walk ten yards along the corridor, and there it was. It took a bit of time, but gradually we got to know each other very well.

Initially, I didn't even know what my new colleagues looked like, as their faces were constantly obscured by PPE. Well, I did know the colour of their eyes and could see the emotion therein, but the rest of their face was a mystery. Facial features isn't really how we get to know someone anyway, it is more about shared emotions. With time we shared feelings of joy (someone going home after making good progress in rehab!), fear (there's been a Covid-19 outbreak in bay three in the ward ... will we get it too? Did I go to bay three last week?), exhaustion (just about everyone at some point had indescribable fatigue), laughter (a 'competition' using a grip strength measurement device to determine who's the 'strongest' clinician on the ward and regularly 'disqualifying' colleagues for the slightest, imagined breaking of the 'competition rules'), and, sadly, not infrequently, burnout (when things became too overwhelming or someone we cared for passed away due to Covid-19). These were difficult times which I am sure left a mark on many health professionals.

Taleb and colleagues (2024) surveyed 1,030 health professionals across 48 countries during the pandemic and found that almost half (49.3%) experienced severe or extremely severe levels of depression, anxiety and stress. Furthermore, almost half (49.6%) experienced burnout. These were all significantly higher than staff who didn't work directly with patients. The factors associated with these adverse psychological experiences being elevated were, as already noted, working directly with patients who had or may have had Covid-19, less previous work experience as a health professional, and having a high workload. It was, of course, not only health professionals who had these experiences. There were many other workers who were essential to ensure the on-going provision of services. For example, those who worked in supermarkets, with extremely high exposure to others *every day. Indeed, a qualitative study conducted during the early stages of the pandemic highlighted how these people also experienced significant anxiety and distress (*May et al., 2021*).*

On a personal level, there were certainly times when I felt utterly drained and depressed by the unrelenting nature of the pandemic. Wonderful colleagues and a strict exercise routine helped to keep that at bay, or at least enough at bay to keep on working in the NHS until the summer of 2021. However, there did come a time when things took a turn for the worse. For the first time in my career, I had to take a few days annual leave after a death that was just the final straw of what, at that time, had started to feel like a never-ending, slowly grinding and creaking conveyor belt of human suffering and despair. It is difficult as a health professional to mourn the loss of someone you knew well as a patient. The first day after they passed away, you feel a shock every time you look at 'their' bed and notice, as if for the first time, that 'the wrong person' is in 'their' bed. A brief moment of 'where are they' and a missed heartbeat inevitably follows, before switching back to what it is you were supposed to be doing. It was clearly time to take a break.

During my first day of leave, my friend and I did a sunset walk on the beach. It was very difficult to put memories of the patient out of my head. I had been ruminating about the three months I knew them in the hospital: the things they said (some funny, some tragic) to me; the look of fear, bewilderment and despair as it became clear that there was no more to be done; coughing and breathing effortfully while I just sat with them in their side room, as a physiotherapist (hopelessly too young to be exposed to such a situation) made a valiant effort to provide some support for their breathing. When I next came to the ward, they were dead. Now whilst walking, reliving these memories, I paused by the waves while my friend continued to walk, becoming smaller and smaller in the distance.

There on my own on the beach, right where the last gasp of the waves barely reach the damp sand before retreating, I packed out the patient's first name in little rounded beach stones. It was the only ceremony to honour their life and passing I could think of in my befuddled mind. Within a short while, the tide would rise and permanently remove the stone symbol of their name. Within a year, I would be out of the NHS, and never (at the time of writing) see my new ward colleagues again, even though I would often think about them and even miss them. The next day, my friend and I walked on the mountains. Looking back, I see I photographed the beautiful light touching the tops of the hills; some in rich colour, many in high contrast black and white. My few days of leave overlapped with my birthday, which cynically made me realise that I would return to duties older (of course) and reflect if that meant wiser too (I don't think so).

A point of note in reflecting on the Taleb et al. (2024) *study:*

On the ward I very briefly describe above, and will explain more later, I have met some of the most remarkable young people ever, including the young physiotherapist I mentioned above. The youth often get a lot of bad press in the media – unfairly so. Some of the young people on my secondment ward had just qualified as clinicians, others were near, or in the final year of their training. None of these people had any previous experience of working independently as a qualified clinician, never mind experience of many years, let alone managing the demands of Covid-19. However, every single one of them were unimaginably brave, committed to working very hard, kind, funny, compassionate, and picked up new skills and knowledge at a ferocious pace. For example, silently offering me, as the oldest member of the clinical team, a chair of sorts to sit on. Or asking if I wanted a coffee when they went to the canteen. It's the small acts of kindness we remember.

Some of these new young colleagues of mine contracted Covid-19 and got very ill. But they returned to the ward. Day after day. I remember walking up the stairs to the isolation ward. While going up the stairs, the young colleague accompanying me fell behind on the staircase and I noticed they were totally out of breath. Upon asking them what was wrong, they looked up at me with defiant, bright young eyes and told me that, despite having been an active runner and into exercise, since they were ill with Covid-19 six months previously, they have not been able to breathe properly (journal entry, October 29, 2020). Their explanation of why they struggled with climbing stairs stunned me, thinking by myself, 'and here you are, going back into an isolation ward with your damaged lungs, selflessly, to help others, under very dangerous conditions'…

(vi) Community Unity: How Can I help?

Lockdown might have sent us all into isolation and kept us within our homes, but that seemed to spark an incredible response from communities across the UK. Strangers reached out to one another across the virtual and real world, making connections and developing innovative approaches to support one another. It was one of the most amazing and positive aspects of those early days of the pandemic where, in the process of shutting ourselves away from everyone, we simultaneously found every possible safe way to reconnect, providing both practical and emotional support to family, friends and reaching a hand out to help those we did not even know.

There has been much written about the critical importance of providing support for people with a brain injury during the pandemic. However, I did not feel that this was a 'one way street' of people supporting me, and my first thoughts were not about what I might need, but rather about what I could do to try to help others. One priority was my elderly neighbour who also lived on his own, far from his family. Even more my concern turned to how I could manage to help my mother, in her 80s, living on her own hundreds of miles away on the other side of the country. Whilst in-person contact and travel had all stopped, I had the power of the internet at my fingers. I soon tapped into the potential of online shopping as a way of getting food sent directly to my mum and ordering food for my neighbour to pass it to him over the garden fence. It was not a straightforward process in those early days, and trying to get one of the limited delivery slots required a 2am alarm to get online as soon as the opportunities were released by various supermarkets.

[Rudi]
*One of my neighbours was a frail, elderly person who
had to shield. They could see me walk past the window
every morning. Initially they looked at me in disbelief
(must have been the scrubs), but soon we exchanged
waves. This progressed to checking every morning with
a thumbs up sign if they were okay after another night
on their own, with their thumb replying everything was
cool. Later, from a distance we started chatting somewhat tentatively, through the window. The usual: how
are you, lovely weather, nasty weather, how are you
today, let me know if you need anything (then what – do
you think it is a good idea for a Covid-19 timebomb to
come into their flat?), or that the world has gone mad,
just look at these politicians.*

*I underestimated what these daily mundane, brief
interactions meant to them. Later, much later, when
contact between neighbours was almost back to normal
and the devastation of the pandemic started to wane
a little bit, they asked me to help them with something
small (but important to them), casually saying that they
'trusted me'. I felt guilty and sad that I had probably
been too emotionally absorbed in the NHS world of
Covid-19 the previous 18 months to be a good friend,
neighbour and member of the community to everyone
around me. Sue beautifully captured in the text above
and below the importance of these acts of kindness waiting to be received by those less fortunate than us, and
living their lives and struggles right next to us.*

I had unfortunately underestimated the cognitive
demands of such a drastic change to my usual routine
of following the same path round the same supermarket

to do my shopping. I ignored the previous experience of the difficulties I had trying to go into alternative shops, where the wrong choices had sent my brain into an over-whelming meltdown. Having a brain injury, especially the issues caused by having a very limited 'working memory' and difficulties with decision making due to executive dysfunction, meant coping with the some-what complicated process of online shopping on behalf of other people taxed my limited cognitive capabilities and significantly increased my neurological fatigue. Trying to manage this provided a useful lesson of the challenges of adapting to this 'new normal' for someone like me with a brain injury.

Although having a brain injury might have limited what I could do, it did not stop the inbuilt desire to support those in need. It is easy to forget that, for some people with a brain injury, their supportive role within their family or social group does not disappear and is often critical to their self-identity. A reduction in cog-nitive capability does not equate to a reduction in car-ing. I found it empowering to be able to help out a little, after feeling increasingly incapable for so long due to my brain injury. It also helped me reconnect with a core aspect of my identity. It was such a strong driver for me to try to help in any way I could as soon as lockdown started, sorting out shopping, checking in with friends, calling family, setting up small online private support groups for people who I knew were liv-ing on their own, and inviting those who I didn't know to join in. My contribution to supporting others was very minor compared to the efforts of so many people, but it felt positive to be able to help even a little bit during this time of crisis.

Communities also united in the initial 'Clap for Carers' – a grassroots initiative that rapidly spread across the country. Although I acknowledged that this expression of gratitude for all key workers was not sufficient to address the challenges of limited PPE and other critical issues, and gave rise to some mixed feelings for care workers themselves (Manthorpe et al., 2022), it felt important to do something to say thank you. It also served an important purpose in bringing communities together.

Sue's Journal March 26, 2020

It was the first 'clap for carers' tonight. I wasn't sure if anyone else would join in or if I'd look a bit daft standing at the doorway clapping on my own. But I figured if I started it here then maybe other people would join in. And they did! It was so poignant, my neighbours slowly emerged, one by one, and it was lovely to see everyone. We could hear not just our own clapping, but the sound of bells ringing and pans banging from across the town. It was so good to see that my neighbours were OK, to have a chat at a distance. It wasn't that long, and then we went back inside. I sat down on the sofa and cried with the mixed emotions of it all. Most of all, I no longer felt so alone.

[Rudi]
I remember the first time hearing the evening 'clap for carers'. At first, I had no idea what it was. The sounds were a visceral mix of clapping and metallic clanging

sound (pots? pans?), but most of all I remember that there was someone playing the drums. I looked out of the window wondering what was going on. Was there a carnival in town to celebrate something I missed? My friend and flatmate, who was more connected to the news and daily events outside of my narrow NHS life, pointed out to me what was happening and suggested we go outside. But I felt too embarrassed and self-conscious to go out to have a look and told her I felt too tired.

As a health professional, it was my duty to do my little bit, which in any case is just my job. Just like the delivery driver who has to get on with delivering parcels, or the Postie making sure we get important mail. And, in any case, my 'Covid-19 tour' was not nearly as intense as those working in Intensive Therapy Units or Accident and Emergency. They deserved the clapping, although it was nowhere near proportional to what they must have gone through and sacrificed. I would have felt very guilty and like a fraud if I went outside to witness the clapping – those who really deserved it were probably at that very moment stuck dehydrated behind PPE, inhaling stale air, seeing critically ill patients for many hours. Other than that first time I have absolutely no memories of the clapping events. I never took any photographs of these events either.

What I remember much more clearly than the 'clap for carers' were the decorations in windows, doors and painted stones on the beach. These were lovely, and I took many, many photographs of the painted stones I encountered in my daily walk by the sea after work. The stones were subtle, tangible little bricks symbolic of the house of community cohesion and taking an interest in the well-being of the ordinary people around us. Two of my favourites were 'Hope' (photographed June 8, 2020) and 'Storms pass' (photographed May 28, 2020). The other thing I remember is the rainbow hearts painted on some of the roads, one in fact on the access road to one of the hospitals where I spent most of my in-patient time (photographed July 5, 2020 – yes, the roads were so quiet I could step into the road to take the picture!).

At first during the early days of the pandemic, the stones were luminous in the spring light; then they gradually faded like many of our memories from the pandemic. Although some memories never went on their way. Speaking of quiet roads, I also remember seeing, to the left through my windscreen, a uniformed hand directing me to turn off the road. My immediate thought was that it served me right for driving (at the time) a red car of a type that just asks to be pulled over by the authorities. Actually, I was being stopped by the Police to (rightly so) ask what the purpose of my journey was. Upon opening the boot of my car to take out my NHS ID and explain why I was on the road, I had a sense that the stash of used PPE visible inside the boot after the day's home visits in the community carried much more weight than my ID in their decision to send me on my way straight away! I am grateful that I kept a journal and took hundreds of photos during the time to help preserve the evidence needed to avoid the personal history from that time to fade, from fact, to fantasy, to forgotten.

This tangible expression of community cohesion, caring and support for those people who were working so hard, and putting themselves at risk, meant a lot to many of us. Along with windows decorated with rainbows, we all wanted to 'do something' to help, to connect with each other, and show our appreciation even in such a small way. Helping out was not just about doing practical things, it was also about supporting our communities and protecting our mental health as well. Like many of the other 'socially distanced' activities that developed during the pandemic, this was also something that I could join in with on an equal basis despite my brain injury and it felt so good to be part of things with everyone else again.

(vii) Daily Exercise: Freedom and Fear

As Rudi notes in his experience of the pandemic, 'daily exercise' became very important to many of us, providing a regular routine. It helped not only our physical cardio-vascular health, but for many of us it also had an impact on our mental health. For me, in those early days, this was a double-edged sword and 'going for a walk' was a mix of both freedom from the confines of my home and fear of encountering other people and the risk of viral transmission even outdoors.

I really appreciated that I was lucky enough to be reasonably protected from the risks of catching the virus, especially compared to key workers – whether that was within a clinical role, such as Rudi, or other essential services, as with my partner. However, I struggled with the confinement of remaining within the same four walls of my small house every day, seemingly without end. I had spent all my life as an active person, hiking and cycling in the mountains outdoors all year and travelling the world for adventure or work. I had always gone out for a walk every day, and even after my accident, my first priority when I had recovered enough was to shuffle ten yards to the nearest bench and sit outside in the fresh air with the assistance of a friend. Now, cooped up in the house during lockdown, I felt like I was going stir-crazy and I just needed to get out.

[Rudi]
For many, engagement in regular recreational exercise became more complicated during the pandemic. Participation in exercise decreased during the pandemic (2021). The environment appeared to play an important role in how, or where, exercise patterns changed. A study published by Rice *et al.* (2020), *during the early days of the pandemic, reported that recreational exercise decreased much more in cities compared to rural areas. Already during the early stages of the pandemic, concerns about the likely negative outcome of sedentary behaviour due to lockdown and reduced opportunities for exercising on cardio-vascular health were raised (Yeo, 2020). Venter et al. (2021) analysed Strava data from 53,000 users and found that, in Norway (Oslo, in particular), during lockdown exercise increased significantly, and was sustained for six months, but moved away from built up inner-city areas towards green spaces. A stark reminder of the importance of green spaces in cities for mental and physical health.*

Strava, other fitness apps and social media allowed some to exercise 'separate but together'. It was possible to 'see', and connect with, friends or family who had been out exercising, and provide social support or encouragement from a safe digital distance. The hills and mountains were deserted, but there were signs of 'life out there', and not always digital. A blue surgical mask stuck in the gorse on the Carneddau, defiantly flapping about in the wind, was a silent reminder that there were other people in the hills, despite the fears around contracting Covid-19 – even outdoors. Being on the mountains was a world as far away as possible for me, which was essential to counter the corrosive effects of the world of the hospital. Data on tracking devices and fitness apps were reinforcing virtual mantras to remind me that eventually everything becomes history. One day during an after-work walk on the beach, I saw a stone among many. But this one was wearing a different coat, not a stony grey, instead spelling out in carefully painted colourful letters that 'storms pass'. It's one of my favourite images from the time.

'Daily Exercise' became my escape route, an opportunity to help both my body and my mind, but it took a lot to begin with to overcome my fears. At the start of lockdown, when so much about Covid-19 was still so unknown, I felt extremely scared of going out at all. In my mind, the virus was 'out there' somewhere, and anyone could have it, or could have left traces of it in other places. The relative lack of knowledge at that point about how it was being transmitted meant that even seeing another person on the street filled me with fear.

Sue's Journal March 30, 2020
  I tried to go out for a walk today, but I got too scared to go far and when I saw someone in the distance I just ran home. I don't know what to do.

Is it safe? There's so much we don't know – all the scientists are saying slightly different things. How far can this virus travel between people, what if someone coughed or shouted nearby? I know about the 'two metre rule' but is this enough, or is that just a guess? I'm also worried about touching something that someone else might have touched recently. They've already told us that it is best to wash some of our shopping, and put the post to one side for three days, but is there a risk of catching the virus if I touched a gate or stile that might have fragments of the virus on it from someone else's hands? How long can the virus stay 'alive' on objects? But I can't face continuing to just stay inside every day.

The discussion on all of these topics was rife with uncertainty. It is easy to forget how little we knew in the first few months of the pandemic and, although these concerns seem exaggerated now, at the time they were very real.

So my first few 'outings' were extremely limited, constrained by fear and anxiety about the virus. I am fortunate that I live in a beautiful rural area, surrounded by beaches, fields, woods and mountains, with few people. To begin with, I just crept out in the early hours at dawn, before anyone else was around, and walked up the little lane at the back of my house through the woods and fields. Worried about the risk of catching the virus from a gate or post that someone else might have touched previously, I used sticks or even small stones as 'gate catch openers' to ensure that I didn't have to touch anything. If nothing else, it improved my balance whilst wobbling over a stile and trying not to use my hands as I climbed over it.

I never saw anyone on my initial dawn walks, but I still had that constant anxiety that something dangerous and threatening was out there hidden somewhere. Although many of us were anxious during this time, I knew in myself that the fear I was feeling was more extreme and was not really an accurate reflection of the level of risk presented by going for a solitary walk outdoors. This fear was a very visceral sensation and was similar to what I had been experiencing on occasions ever since my accident.

[Rudi]
Very similar to Sue, I was aware that there was 'something in the air'. In the hospital environment this was obvious – hospitals, after all, have their own signature smell – but strangely enough, during work this awareness only occasionally came to consciousness. For example, more so when seeing a patient in a hot ward or bay, or in a stuffy side room. It was outside of the hospital where this became more of a thing. In a supermarket, 'there's a lot of breathing here, what's in the air...?', or when refuelling, 'how many people have already handled the fuel hose today, were their hands clean...?'. These types of thoughts, completely unannounced, drifting into my consciousness, before silently, without providing an answer, leaving my consciousness again. I guess some of these silent inner dialogues may have made some of us look a bit distracted or even tired. Which, of course, we were. I certainly was, and sometimes caught myself not quite registering what someone was saying

With the focus on the impairments due to my brain injury, I had not registered that the first word of my type of injury was 'traumatic'. Nor did I realise the legacy that this would leave and the impact that it would have on my response to the pandemic, particularly feelings of threat, fear and anxiety. These emotions were exacerbated by some of my cognitive impairments; in particular, my slow speed of processing and limited working memory meant that I was extremely nervous of 'missing something' that could cause me harm, often rendering me unable to move. I would stand on the kerb beside the road, or near the edge of a driveway, desperately trying to look every way, but as soon as I turned my head, I would be frantically thinking that I had forgotten where I just looked and I would freeze with fear. With the arrival of Covid-19, this terror didn't just apply to roads and driveways anymore. Now it had extended and it felt like the 'threat' could be anywhere out there.

My fear of going out had started after the car had hit me, in a way that I didn't understand and couldn't explain. Although the fact that the car had appeared suddenly, seemingly out of nowhere, probably sits behind much of my subsequent anxiety. Having such a terrible accident happen to me that I couldn't anticipate or prevent really made me feel extremely worried about 'bad things' happening to me again. For the first time in my life, I felt so vulnerable, psychologically shrinking inside myself, trying to protect myself from unexpected harm. Before the pandemic, even in the most innocuous of normal everyday situations, an unexpected 'trigger' would cause me to psychologically cower and flinch, and physically my shoulders would hunch, arms tucked it, trying to get as small as possible to protect myself from a feeling of impact. I'd freeze in fear, biting my lip, digging in my nails, trying to keep control and not run away like a demented thing. Without realising it, I was experiencing 'flashbacks' on a regular basis from my accident. I had thought flashbacks would be like a memory of the event that was replayed in the current time, but what I experienced was more like real-time sensations of absolute terror, instinctual reactions, and a certain expectation of imminent impact and death. Most of all, in that immediate moment I experienced the unmistakable metallic taste and smell of blood, even though at this point nothing was bleeding. It was the same visceral experience I had when I hit the car and when I felt I was going to die from drowning in my own blood. I had an unconscious feeling of overwhelming sensations and terror in those few moments when I expected death, and I felt that I was reliving these over and over again. When these experiences returned at times after my accident, I was not reliving the past. Instead, these felt like real sensations in current time and instinctively I did all I could to protect myself, even though now there was no real harm in front of me.

[Rudi]
Post-traumatic stress disorder (PTSD), or features of PTSD, are common after traumatic brain injury, and even more so where loss of consciousness was not complete and patients have 'islands of memory' around the event where they sustained their injury (Howlett, Nelson & Stein, 2022). Furthermore, in my clinical experience it is also not uncommon for many different types of associative stimuli to trigger the anxiety and other symptoms of PTSD. What that means it that something

that was emotionally highly arousing during an event is more likely to be remembered or associated with said event. Examples include the smell of petrol being associated with a road traffic collision where a driver was trapped whilst there was a risk of fire. Therefore, when the person fills up their car, symptoms are triggered unexpectedly. Or the sound of an overhead jet howling through the air above a combatant exposed to bombing. Another example is the sound of an ambulance siren or hospital smell when a pedestrian run over by a car is subsequently exposed to these perceptual stimuli.

Triggers can, over time, generalise, with similar or related stimuli to the original now re-triggering PTSD symptoms. In an interesting long-term study of veterans previously diagnosed with PTSD, Solomon et al. (2021) found that Covid-19 and all the anxiety associated with it made these veterans more at risk to re-experience PTSD, an intensification of symptoms or relapses. It is often the case that the unexpected or 'out of the blue' nature of the event which resulted in a person's injury in itself becomes a trigger. What that means in simple language is that people with PTSD find the potential for experiencing 'unpleasant surprises' very difficult. They also experience 'the unknown' as very stressful – a situation arises where there may be danger, but it is not known what that might be.

Although I had experienced these flashbacks of sensations a lot in the first few months since my accident, it had subsided as time passed. But now, with the threat of the pandemic, it was back with a vengeance. For some reason, my brain had now attached the risk of the virus to my fear of getting hit by a car and the visceral memories I had from my accident. Now a person appearing suddenly who might have the virus was as terrifying to me as a car emerging from a hidden driveway. To my brain, it did not matter if the threat was a car or a person who potentially had the virus, my physical and psychological response was the same: uncontrollable fear and an overwhelming urge to protect myself, as if I was again facing death itself in that moment. The strong repeated warnings in the daily national news of 'anyone can catch it', the tragic images of people struggling to breathe in hospitals, the red and white warning tape and signs cutting off car parks and shops, and the police patrolling the roads, all combined to elevate that fear and the level of risk in my mind. Like a red alert, the warning lights were constantly flashing in my brain, saying 'danger', 'danger' over and over again. I felt it when I went out for my little walks, beside driveways and hedges, at road junctions, and anywhere else where an 'unseen threat' might appear. In particular, the mere thought of even seeing another person in the far distance provoked this reaction. It would leave me shaking and nauseous, and I would 'feel' the sensation of terror, impact and pain, even though there was nothing happening to me. I couldn't stop it, and I couldn't control it.

The more I tried to manage and suppress this panic, the more it pervaded my dreams. Horrific nightmares were a regular occurrence, full of terrifying gruesome injuries, pain and suffering, in all of which I was powerless to avoid getting hurt, unable to stop or prevent it from happening. I became scared of what was happening in my own head. What if the accident and damage to my brain had changed me into someone who was potentially dangerous and I might cause harm to myself or others? Would I get locked up or put away in an institution?

For a long time, I was too frightened to even talk about it to anyone. It took a lot of trust to finally share some of these nightmares and 'flashbacks' with Rudi in my rehabilitation sessions. To speak of the darkest corners of our minds is to reveal a level of vulnerability to another person, and Rudi's sensitivity in explaining these nightmares and the process by which traumatic memories recur as flashbacks was greatly appreciated. Learning a bit more about how trauma is not properly processed as a 'memory' really helped me to understand more about what was happening. I was fully conscious and hyper alert in the few seconds before my accident, but unconscious after the impact, with subsequent periods of alternating consciousness and post-traumatic amnesia for several weeks. This meant I had both conscious memories of the actual event, and somatic memories which recalled the smells and sounds of my experience, even though I had no conscious knowledge of these things happening. If I had experienced a total lack of consciousness, then the resulting loss of memories would have had a protective effect.

The UK brain injury charity, Headway (2020), notes the relationship between a traumatic brain injury and post-traumatic stress disorder, along with other significant anxiety issues. Exploring this in more detail has helped me realise that these flashbacks and my heightened level of anxiety regarding perceived threat was not just 'all in my mind' but was related to specific memory processing issues from my accident. There is some discussion about whether the cognitive effects of a TBI increase the prevalence of PTSD, or whether these issues of stress and flashbacks are purely related to the effect of a highly traumatic experience. A comprehensive, systematic review of this relationship was undertaken by Van Praag et al. (2019) and found to be a complex picture:

> Several studies compared PTSD rates between patients with a TBI with non-brain injury trauma patients ... Meta-analysis across these studies did reveal a higher prevalence of PTSD in patients with TBI. This lends some support to the concept that TBI-specific factors, such as disruption in brain circuitry, may underlie the comorbidity of TBI and PTSD. The high heterogeneity between studies, however, prevents drawing strong conclusions. ... The association between PTSD symptoms and TBI is complex: the lack of a clear association between TBI severity and prevalence of PTSD raises the question of to what extent the brain injury itself plays a role in the development of PTSD and how the brain injury might affect the course of PTSD. How do consequences of TBI, such as cognitive deficiencies or problematic social re-integration interfere with PTSD and its treatment? Future research needs to focus on the event itself; pre-trauma- and patient-related factors, for example, personality factors; and post-trauma setting, for example, social support, taking into account the specific symptoms of TBI and its consequences.
>
> (Van Praag et al., 2019)

My experience of heightened anxiety and flashbacks, which got much worse during the pandemic, could be an example of the impact of events in this 'post-trauma' period. I do not know what would have been the situation if Covid-19, with all its associated warnings and risks, had not come along within the first 18 months after my traumatic accident while I was going through the early stages of my brain injury rehabilitation. Would my flashbacks have reduced, or would this heightened state of anxiety have continued anyway?

Trying to understand my 'triggers' for these flashbacks and nightmares was a bit more complex. Some were easy for me to comprehend – hidden driveways, road junctions, the flash of the colour red at the corner of my vision. These all had a direct connection to the events of my accident. However, it is only with the benefit of hindsight that I now recognise how much the messages about the threat of the virus acted as a trigger for me. Watching the news on the TV every day meant that I constantly heard strongly worded official voices repeating the danger of this 'unsee-able threat' which 'anyone can have' and 'anyone can pass on', along with the phrase 'stay safe, stay at home, save lives'. Like a homing pigeon, my brain focused on these aspects of the threat of the virus, and Covid-19 – or rather, the people who might be carrying it, who to me was potentially anyone – became like an overwhelming 'trigger' in my mind. So the risk of encountering people, even out on my walks, caused the same sensations and flashbacks as my other triggers now.

Therefore, it was not surprising that going out for my 'daily exercise' was initially a conflicting mix of fear and freedom. However, as the first lockdown continued, my urge to get out grew stronger and I began to develop strategies that helped me to overcome these fears. In doing so, these approaches not only reduced my stress levels and fear-based flashbacks, but I slowly realised that they were also simultaneously helping me manage some of the cognitive impairments of my brain injury.

(viii) Photography: Focusing my Mind

In an attempt to persuade myself to go out and manage this fear in the early days of lockdown, I set myself a project. I started taking daily photos, returning to my previous love of photography in the outdoors. In March and April 2020, it was early spring and the first leaves were unfurling in the trees along with small buds of wildflowers emerging in the hedgerows, woods and fields. Going out on my little walks with my camera, I focused (literally and metaphorically) on capturing close-up images of these wonderful wildflowers. I would stop for ages on my knees, admiring a single flower and its delicate intricate colours, waiting poised for the breeze to pause for a fraction of a second so I could capture a focused photo. Inevitably, I would get tempted further up the path, seeing a new flower emerging, encouraging me to go out on longer walks. Soon I added the challenge of capturing close-up photos of busy bumblebees and stunning butterflies requiring even greater concentration and focus. These elements of nature also served another purpose. Despite being so limited in where I could go for a walk and just doing the same route every day, I found that I was still able to experience change and diversity. Instead of travelling to different places to see new things, I found that if I stayed in the same place that nature would ensure that the world would change around me. New flowers appeared, landscapes changed from a muddy brown to grassy fields, and the skeleton branches of winter trees regrew with the electric green of new leaves. I greatly appreciated seeing something new every day and became much more mindful of the changes of emerging spring. In contrast to my previous, pre-brain injury life, when I was always rushing from one place to another, now I was learning the value of staying still and letting change occur around me.

[Rudi]
Photography is a wonderful activity to 'be in the moment', and observe the things around us. In this context, as a therapeutic activity, it can make a contribution to rehabilitation after brain injury. A study by Lorenz (2012) included 13 participants and explored more than 500 photographs to learn more about the therapeutic self-expression and sense making of persons who had suffered a brain injury. Photography also has the potential to complement psychotherapeutic work after brain injury; in particular, around the themes of loss, awareness and meaning (Coetzer, 2015). Photography is a creative activity, but there are also the more 'hidden' ecologically valid benefits of cognitive stimulation and aspects of taking photographs being similar to some elements of mindfulness.

During the pandemic, I took hundreds and hundreds of photographs; sometimes of things very pandemic-related, but not necessarily always. While taking photographs directly related to the pandemic was possibly my personal attempt to make sense of and remember what could potentially quickly be suppressed and deliberately forgotten, those that were not had a different function. I have taken photographs since my early university years and later, after qualifying as a clinician, went to art school part-time for three years to study photography. Looking back now, I must have done that as an escape from the emotional demands of working as a neuropsychologist in an under-resourced state hospital located in a very deprived area with endless numbers of patients who were victims of violence, poverty and disease of an unimaginable scale. The beauty of art is an antidote to witnessing the results of human suffering every day.

During the pandemic, for me photographs of 'ordinary' things in nature, took on a particular beauty, a reminder that life (and the world) has been around for a very long time; chapters pass, new life is created, and one day, who knows, things may be 'normal' again. One the other hand, my pandemic photos were my evidence of being there in what often felt like something I wasn't really part of, just a movie I was watching from a safe distance. A Netflix production I saw, a spectator of sorts of an unfolding disaster movie. But I wasn't a spectator. The photographs were entry visas to the world of Covid-19, and a 'it really happened, and I was there' stamp in my pandemic passport. Other photos, for example of the beautiful wild ponies of the Carneddau, or the desolate landscape they live in, were the psychological exit visas out of the bleak world of Covid-19. These photos brought peace, solace, and escape.

Photographs also capture epochs. A vivid colour photograph I took of a glorious rainbow outside of the hospital (where I did most of my ward work) on. October 30, 2020 (at the end of month seven of the pandemic) has a note 'air, hope, love, water' underneath it. A month later (November 27), there is a bleak, black and white photograph of the mountains with a thin line of sunshine illuminating the darkness and shadows. The non-pandemic personal highlight of the first month of 2021 is captured in a series of photos of a dog lost in bitter cold in the snow overnight on the mountains. The dog appeared out of nowhere while I was walking with my friend, hypothermic, exhausted and needing to be rewarmed and carried down. For the record, she gulped down my hot tea, was extremely heavy to carry in the snow, and difficult to grip whilst wrapped in my emergency foil – and overjoyed, as well as miraculously revived upon seeing her owner not too long after! The small, beautiful events of life, despite the awfulness of the pandemic, still happened. I am now very grateful to have these and many other photos of that time.

What about portraits, or 'selfies', during the pandemic? An interesting study by George et al. (2021) looked at doctors in PPE using a self-portrait stuck to their PPE to facilitate communication with patients. The study found that both doctors and patients found this very helpful and that there were clear psychological benefits to being able to 'see' who's behind the mask (George et al., 2021). Returning to the photographs I took during the pandemic, scrolling through hundreds of pictures, suddenly a self-portrait stares back at me, looking stubbled and exhausted. Coffee in hand, in blue scrubs, mask drawn down, standing in front of a hand-washing station. The lighting looks slightly yellow, like illness starting to reveal itself. The date and time on the metadata of this photo says it was taken October 29, 2020, 22:05. It's the day my young colleague, with what now certainly sounds like Long Covid, struggled to climb the stairs on our way to see patients on the isolation ward.

An old cliché springs to mind: every picture tells a story. A selfie taken February 25, 2021 at 12:16 shows me smiling, in purple scrubs, mask down, holding a small card. Zooming in on the card, it is a vaccination card, with my second shot of Pfizer administered that morning duly recorded. Whilst waiting, I met a doctor who I peripherally knew from the past and we chatted for a bit while waiting our turn. He looked a lot thinner than I remembered him; it transpired they were very ill during the early stage of the pandemic but eventually managed to return to work. February 25 became a very long day and I suspect I became increasingly dehydrated. Either that, or I had a reaction to the second vaccination (the first was okay). According to my friend, at around 03:00 on February 26, I had collapsed on my way to the bathroom. I don't have any memory of that. My friend said the coldness of the floor made me come to again. My dairy says later that day (a Friday) I worked in the ward. My memories of that shift is like looking at a distant scene through a glass bottle roughened up by the sea.

I also found a form of 'companionship' in my shadow, capturing images of myself as a long-legged dark form over the golden sands of my local beach. I much preferred my shadow to the more popular 'selfie'; in part because the evening light of the low sun created an elongated shadow which made me look a bit taller and thinner! My 'shadow photos' were also a very tangible, visual reminder of the isolation of lockdown, as I would go for my daily walk on my own so the only pictures of people that I could take were of 'me'. I would compare these images with my 'pre-pandemic' and 'pre-brain injury' photos, which were always full of the happy, laughing faces of my family and friends.

I found this concentration on taking photos, considering their composition, light, and close-up detail, helped to reduce my fear as I focused completely on something else rather than my anxieties. To my surprise, I did not find that taking photos tired my brain in the same way as other cognitively demanding activities. Instead, 'focusing on just one thing' seemed to help by reducing the external and internal distractions that required so much brain power for me now to manage. I started to learn that despite my many cognitive impairments, my brain actually did quite well when I concentrated on just one thing. As part of my 'lockdown project', I decided to create a photobook to document this strange time. This really helped me fill some of the emptiness of lockdown. Unable to work due to the effects of my brain injury, and with extremely limited opportunities to do anything or go anywhere, along with the isolation of not being able to see anyone, I struggled with the seemingly endless days. My photobook became a long-term goal which helped add a sense of purpose to my days and I concentrated on improving my skills and technique. Photography soon became part of my approach to rehabilitation, and it is a self-management technique that I continue to use to this day.

Research into brain injury rehabilitation is increasingly taking note of the role of creative arts, including photography. There are potentially multiple benefits, including improving concentration and attention, relieving symptoms of anxiety and depression, assisting with self-management and improving self-esteem. More recent developments have explored the importance of creative arts therapy in rehabilitation for people with a traumatic brain injury and co-occurring PTSD (Levy et al., 2025).

Further studies have been done on the importance of photography as a therapeutic intervention to help with coping with the mental health impacts of Covid- 19. A study by Burton and Elliot (2023) reviewed the impact of a photo-reflection intervention on the subjective well-being of participants during the pandemic. Although this study was based on the general population, its findings could be applied equally to people with a brain injury, as well as clinicians – such as Rudi working within the NHS, who also reflects on his practice of taking photos during the pandemic. The benefits of purposeful photography in the aforementioned study included: acting as a prompt for people to plan and undertake positive activities; a coping mechanism to improve well-being during lockdown; as well as useful in therapist–client practices. Burton and Elliot (2023) note that the wider evidence base shows that the self-directed process of taking photographs for therapeutic purposes also has benefits:

> Research has shown that self-guided photography interventions can have positive impacts. An ethnographic study by Brewster and Cox (2019) used observation and interviews to explore the experiences of individuals committed to taking a 'photo-a-day' and sharing this on social media. The interaction with online communities enhanced well-being for some, however the process of photography itself,

through creativity and being mindful of daily events was experienced as a form of self-care with the potential to enhance well-being. Chen et al. (2016) also explored the value of photography for promoting positive affect ... Happiness increased across all conditions and interview data indicated that those taking photographs for their own affect reported becoming more reflective, while those taking photos to send to others found the connection with family and friends helped to relieve stress.

(Burton & Elliot, 2023)

Interestingly, although the research in these studies is based on the experience of the general population, the benefits of photography for certain cognitive functions are also noted:

There is evidence that photo-taking modulates attentional processes and memory accuracy (Henkel, 2014), increases experiential engagement (Diehl et al., 2016) and potentially provides a protective coping effect to mental health in traumatic environments (Feinstein et al., 2020; Ramirez et al., 2019).

(Burton & Elliot, 2023)

For someone like myself with a brain injury, especially with attentional and memory impairment, it felt like my 'daily photos' helped me manage my brain injury as well as my mental health. However, ultimately these self-guided approaches to my brain injury were not sufficient and I was extremely grateful to have the clinical support of Rudi as part of my neurorehabilitation during the lockdown and the challenges of the pandemic.

(ix) The Benefit of Nature

Going outside and enjoying nature, whether that was in the garden, park or wider countryside, was something that many of us valued during the first lockdown. I have always enjoyed being out in the mountains and beside the sea, and it was something that I found particularly beneficial after I had my brain injury. There is something intrinsically valuable about being in nature and there is an extensive evidence base on the mental health benefits of this experience. Whilst this applies to everyone, there is potentially an added value from nature for people with a brain injury. Headway (2020) notes that research has shown that nature-based rehabilitation after brain injury can help with motivation, mood, emotional regulation, sensory motor and cognitive functions. This was substantiated by a scoping review of nature-based rehabilitation for adults with an acquired brain injury (ABI), where a comprehensive systematic analysis of numerous studies concluded:

> Results suggest that nature-based rehabilitation may benefit individuals with acquired brain injury, as both motor – and sensory-motor functions, as well as cognitive functions were significantly improved. Furthermore, two studies found an improvement in quality of life.
>
> (Vibholm et al., 2020)

I felt this benefit after my accident when, even in the early days, I found respite in the peaceful woods and hills by my house. Just sitting quietly in green spaces, with a gentle breeze, and the sound of the birds felt restorative.

To me, this was more than just 'feeling better', which many of us probably experience in such peaceful, natural surroundings. Something was happening in my brain. My cognitive functions felt like they had more capability and had improved more than if I had rested in a similar way indoors. Why was this? It was something that I found difficult to articulate or explain.

As a researcher who specialises in the health benefits of the environment, I looked into the scientific evidence to see if there was a possible explanation for what I was experiencing. In particular, how did being in nature help to improve my cognitive functions? What was the mechanism which was acting as the pathway for this relationship between nature and my brain?

Attention Restoration Theory (ART) (Kaplan, 1989) offers some insight into this, and suggests that, in all people, the ability to concentrate can be improved through exposure to natural environments. ART benefits 'directed attention' – the cognitive capacity to focus on an activity, even in a situation where there are more interesting distractions. This requires effort and can therefore result in attention fatigue.

> ART proposes that individuals benefit from the chance to (1) "be away" from everyday stresses, (2) experience expansive spaces and contexts ("extent"), (3) engage in activities that are "compatible" with our intrinsic motivations, and (4) critically experience stimuli that are "softly fascinating" (Kaplan, 1995). This combination of factors encourages "involuntary" or "indirect attention" and enables our "voluntary" or "directed" attention capacities to recover and restore …. Relaxing settings (such as places of

worship) and activities (such as sleep) may provide restorative opportunities, but ART argues that nature may be particularly useful because it has an "aesthetic advantage" .... It is suggested that spending time in the natural world allows individuals the opportunity for "reflection" and consideration of unresolved issues.

(Ohly et al., 2016)

However, there is still a lack of robust empirical evidence on ART, and the systematic review undertaken by Ohly et al. (2016) found mixed results:

Meta-analyses provided some support for ART, with significant positive effects of exposure to natural environments for three measures (Digit Span Forward, Digit Span Backward, and Trail Making Test B). The remaining 10 meta-analyses did not show marked beneficial effects ... There is uncertainty regarding which aspects of attention may be affected by exposure to natural environments.

(Ohly et al., 2016)

Whilst the evidence regarding ART might be relatively inconclusive, it is notable to me that these studies involved the general population. There remains a question concerning the benefit of exposure to nature for people with a clinical attention deficit, including those of us with a traumatic brain injury. As I discussed previously, there are several different types of attention, and it might be that my lived experience of the restorative effects of greenspace on my cognitive functions is related to the specific attention difficulties that I have from my type of brain injury.

A recent, rigorous randomised control trial (RCT) explored the potential benefits of nature for people with a brain injury. Based on a direct comparison of a walk in nature versus the equivalent walk in an urban area, this research used both self-reported mood responses (affect) and, most interestingly, electroencephalography (EEG) data to examine the effect on executive functions in the brain.

> Behavioural studies suggest that immersion in nature improves affect and executive attention ... While affect improved for both groups, the nature walkers showed a significantly greater boost in positive affect than the urban walkers. Electroencephalography (EEG) data revealed significantly greater FMθ activity following the urban walk compared to the nature walk, suggesting that the urban walk placed higher demands on executive attention. In contrast, the nature walk allowed executive attention to rest, as indicated by the lower FMθ activity observed after the walk. This study suggests that changes in FMθ may be a potential neural mechanism underlying the attentional strain of urban environments in contrast to the attentional rest in nature.
>
> (McDonnel & Strayer, 2024)

Given the number of people with a brain injury who experience benefits from being in natural places, this is something that would be interesting to explore further. Certainly, based on my lived experience there is an additional cognitive improvement from walking or sitting in green spaces. The restrictions of the Covid-19 pandemic, which led many of us to have a more 'outdoor' life, might lead to greater insights for new approaches to neurorehabilitation.

So my 'daily exercise' of walks in the woods and hills during lockdown benefited my brain injury rehabilitation due to being in nature. Based on my experience, I felt that it helped to increase my cognitive capacity and improve my attentional abilities, which in turn reduced my neurological fatigue.

[Rudi]
Above, Sue provides an excellent review of the literature around the benefits of exercise, as well as providing a truly unique insight into this through her lived experience. Walking outside, often in the mountains, was the perfect escape for me too. Whilst out there, it was as if there was no pandemic, just vast open landscape, a million miles away from the hospital. Every single day from late March 2020 I went outside and walked. By the end of the first year of the pandemic, the benefits of being in nature were not only a well-formed habit, but also compelled me to, like with the photographs, more systematically 'document' to remind myself that I didn't imagine it, it really happened. Almost like a frantic attempt to irrevocably 'save' these memories before they have a chance to fade into the obscurity of forgetting who we were during the pandemic. After a technology setback or two, from January 1, 2021, I started to GPS record all outdoor physical activities.

My own phenomenological experience of being in nature also almost exactly mirrors that of Sue. Moving, outside, often in nature, every day, no matter what, probably was the singularly most psychologically protective thing I could do for myself. Exercising was the

one thing I could do to ensure that I was as well as pos-
sible to be able to pitch up for work every day, and do
my best to help those who were often not able anymore
to enjoy the freedom of moving outside. This new habit
of doing some form of exercise outside is one of the good
things that came out of the pandemic for me. The other
thing was talking. It's difficult to talk to someone about
things you'd rather forget. But walking, running, or hik-
ing outside makes that easier. According to Strava, my
friend and I moved outside together, often in beautiful
Snowdonia, for thousands of kilometers since 2020, but
the app's GPS data of course doesn't capture the thou-
sands of conversations we had whilst doing that.

(x) Return to Rehab: Talking on the Phone

I was not at all surprised at the start of lockdown to
get a letter from the North Wales Brain Injury Service
saying that in-person appointments had stopped due to
the virus. It was a completely correct decision, taking
account of the risk to both staff and patients, and in my
mind it was appropriate given the huge ask that was
now being made of all staff in the NHS. I felt extremely
guilty at the mere thought of taking up precious medical resources at this time for what I perceived as the
much lesser issue of my brain injury. People across the
world were dealing with an awful virus for which there
was little treatment and terrible consequences, and there
was a strong narrative amongst my social peers of not
doing anything that would add to the demands on the
NHS. Knowing the scale of the challenge that was faced
by the health service, I felt completely undeserving of

any continuing support for my brain injury. This guilt of using up precious resources, and being unworthy of treatment, has long been an aspect of my feelings about my rehabilitation. Significantly exacerbated by the pandemic, it also compounded some of the intrinsic challenges I faced in adjusting my self-identity from feeling like a 'strong' person who is always there to help others, to negative self-perceptions as someone whose brain injury makes me 'weak' and in need of support.

However, at the same time, I felt my ability to cope with my brain injury was deteriorating significantly; in part due to the impact of the pandemic. I had only just started the process of beginning to understand my cognitive impairments and had not really begun the long journey of accepting that I was not going to 'get better' and that I would need to adjust in order to accommodate and manage the effects of my brain injury. So a sudden stop to my rehabilitation, at such an early stage after over a year of trying and failing to cope, felt like being dropped back into a world of confusion. In addition, the sudden restrictions of the lockdown caused significant changes to all my routines, along with the removal of practical and social support, which combined to increase my anxiety and neurological fatigue.

[Rudi]
At the very start of the pandemic, we were apprehensive about how to care for our existing patients now that in-person appointments were deemed not possible. Too little knowledge about risk of transmission, individual vulnerability to severe illness, and a multitude of other factors, made an informed decision based on evidence and science almost impossible at this stage. It was one

of the most difficult decisions I have ever made as a health professional, but the 'ethical', 'moral', 'heart', and 'pragmatism', all combined to come up with a solution, which was a hybrid model. We would start with making contact with our patients by letter or telephone and put in place a triage system of 'who needs what, when, and how'. Furthermore, appointments could be digital, or where clinically indicated, in-person. Finally, when the time came for some of us to do in-person clinical work in the wards we used to cover, as well as the new isolation wards, the allocation was to be via voluntary secondment to these hospitals and units based on their needs. That was our plan to try and as far as possible minimise the disruption in rehabilitation for persons 'already on the books', as well as new referrals.

I was not alone in facing these issues. A national survey undertaken by Headway in the first year of the pandemic (2020) found that 57% of people who sustained their brain injury in the last two years said that their access to specialist treatment had been negatively impacted. Like me, this was worse for people in the earlier stages of their rehabilitation journey, especially with the detrimental effects of continuing Covid-19 restrictions which were expected to be on-going:

Face-to-face rehabilitation is likely to continue to be restricted for some time. This is concerning as the first two years following a brain injury are very important in terms of a patient's long-term prognosis and any delay to receiving specialist rehabilitation can impact their ability to lead an independent life in the future.

(Headway, 2020)

Like a lifeline into this darkness, I was extremely grateful when the North Wales Brain Injury Service contacted me to offer a phone appointment with Rudi to check in and continue my rehabilitation. I am fully aware of how fortunate I was to have this opportunity. Even in these early days of the pandemic, the negative impacts of not having access to neurorehabilitation had prompted a shift to telehealth approaches in community-based neuropsychological rehabilitation, not just for me but for many people with a brain injury both in the UK and other countries. The long-term nature of rehabilitation, combined with the on-going restrictions of lockdown, meant that a 'one-off check-in call' was not going to be sufficient and there would need to be a more systematic shift to telehealth approaches, and the urgency of this was noted in the early response to rehabilitation during the pandemic in Italy:

> To be effective, cognitive rehabilitation programs must be intensive and prolonged over time; however, the current virus containment measures are hampering their implementation. Moreover, the reduced access to cognitive rehabilitation might worsen the relationship between the patient and the healthcare professional. Urgent measures to address issues connected to COVID-19 pandemic are, therefore, needed. Remote communication technologies are increasingly regarded as potential effective options to support health care interventions, including neurorehabilitation and cognitive rehabilitation.
> (Mantovani et al., 2020)

The initial phone calls with Rudi felt strange and difficult to adjust to after having previously had in-person

discussions at the clinic. There were a few techno-
logical glitches which made connecting a somewhat
haphazard process at times, frustrating for both of us
on each end of the line as repeated attempts were made
to 'dial in'. These technical challenges brought with
them greater cognitive demands, trying to remember
the right numbers and process. On the phone, a disem-
bodied voice replaced the more familiar contact of in-
person appointments, and in particular a 'friendly face'.
I found it difficult to communicate initially beyond
more factual information, and these discussions were
in the first instance a more transactional exchange
than an insightful interaction. Losing the opportunity
to see non-verbal cues removed the subtleties of more
nuanced and detailed communication. Since my brain
injury, I had lost my previous instinctual ability to
both think and speak as a seamless process, which was
replaced by a more stuttering and slower approach to
direct conversation. So I had to rely on doing my 'thinking' before my rehab sessions, writing my key points
onto a piece of paper to discuss with Rudi at the clinic.
That paper on the table also served as an opportunity
for mid-discussion drawing of things that I could not
find the words to explain, relying on analogies and sim-
iles. This rich, complex, verbal and visual multi-modal
communication could not be reproduced in a telephone
discussion.

Qualitative studies based on interviews with people
with an acquired brain injury have also found that many
felt there were numerous benefits relating to connection and multi-dimensional interaction from in-person
rehabilitation which were not so easily transferred to a
phone call:

Overall, a preference for in-person care was widely noted, because of its ability to embody the essence of human interaction. The following sentences describe that 'essence', which includes feeling seen, supported, and connected with one another. Participants craved in-person interactions with peers and healthcare professionals, as they have provided an immense amount of support during their recovery ... The multidimensional nature of rehabilitation emphasizes how in-person therapy results in better healing, learning, and outcomes.

(Wong et al., 2022)

[Rudi]
Making telephone calls has never been my favourite thing, and even less so in a healthcare setting. A very late adopter of smartphones, I prefer to avoid phones, mobile or landline. Like brown envelopes in your in-tray, unexpected phone calls hardly ever contain any good news. But now with the unexpected outbreak of a pandemic, and especially initially when very little was known for certain about the virus and its transmission, we had to find pragmatic ways to adjust our practice to protect our patients. Probably the worst fear as a health professional is that you will accidently and unintentionally harm a patient in any way. A time to let go of the luxury of preference then. Phones will have to become my (hopefully short-term!) friend. With that started the first attempts to re-establish input to people already in our care, and where a referral letter deemed it safe to do an initial telephone screening before deciding to see the patient in person, or not. At least in that way some sort

of quick triage system for new referrals, and the lifeline of re-establishing contact with existing patients, could be put in place with minimal disruption.

This is how it came about that whilst sitting at my desk in my tiny NHS office reserved really only for writing clinical notes, I heard the brief sound of an electronic connection being established, and the phone being answered. The brief doubt of 'did I dial the correct number' during the first second of silence, before an electronically altered voice of a person answered. Then followed a couple of seconds of intense information processing before the 'internal clearance to proceed' and mental connection of 'yes, that's Sue's voice' was made in my mind. I remember closing my eyes in a desperate attempt to have at least some 'visual processing channel' available to me, but of course that only called up historical images. The information processing load can be considerable when making telephone calls in a clinical context. For me, anyway, it was. Nevertheless, it was a relief to re-establish contact with Sue and, despite the limitations of having only auditory processing available, it felt good to make the initial contact that would inevitably be needed to, with time, continue the work Sue and I had been doing at the unit.

From my personal perspective, providing clinical input via telephone was hard work and less than ideal. But putting that aside, what are the views of patients? It is interesting to note that patient preference (or not) for telephone, or other means of remote healthcare contact, is not universally the same for everyone. Tyerman *et al.* (2021) *conducted a survey of 58 people with acquired brain injury and obtained information about how they experienced remote contact. Their findings were that patients had a range of experiences to remote contact, with most preferring a flexible balance between face-to-face and remote, while a third preferred face-to-face. Interestingly, there was a strong suggestion that patients in their first year post-injury found remote clinical contact more difficult, expressing a preference for in-person care. That mirrors my own personal experience of providing care during the pandemic. While many of our patients (the majority as far as I recall) were very grateful for the in-person community home visits, a fair proportion were actually relieved we mutually agreed not to do that and instead work remotely, or alternatively, wait 'for a better time'.*

(xi) Hospitals: Neurorehabilitation on the Wards

In contrast to the relatively minor practical issues of telephone treatment, Rudi faced the much more significant challenge of returning to treat people in hospital. This is his personal lived experience of the issues he faced working at the hospital during the initial period of the pandemic.

[Rudi] March 30, 2020
I am back at work, inside the NHS community hospital where our service is located and where I have worked for almost 20 years as a consultant neuropsychologist by now. Clearly, I know the place well, but it feels surreal to be inside a hospital, now, of all places. Outside history unfolds by the day, changing society as we knew it. Over the next 18 months a reflective journal ('the conference freebie blue A5 notebook') and many, many

photographs, will help me to remember, to capture, to preserve, and perhaps one day make some sense of the pandemic once it is history. For now, though, back in the hospital where I am based, a few early strategies to support our patients, including sending letters, and making contact via telephone, has to be put in place. The usual hustle and bustle of a busy community out-patient neurorehabilitation unit has died down, replaced by muted telephone conversations from behind closed clinic room doors. Occasionally, we briefly see each other walking in the passage or silently grabbing a coffee in the kitchen.

A few weeks later, myself and three other colleagues in our service voluntarily second to the hospital wards to work in-person, where persons with acquired brain injury are cared for and receiving rehabilitation. Two I know well, having been colleagues in the service for more than a decade. But the third person's volunteering touches my heart very deeply. The third volunteer is my trainee on clinical placement with me. Please don't let them get sick, or worse. To this day, I think of them and their choice to second during the pandemic, which was the opposite of the majority. A minority decision by them to do something truly remarkable, brave, kind and selfless, potentially a missed opportunity for many. A pandemic increases the need for psychological care, the presence of another human, being able to <u>talk</u> about your fears and other feelings, to someone who is there by your side. If ever there was a time in history for the 'talking' therapies, this was it. A pandemic does not take away the risks of sustaining a traumatic brain injury, suffering a Stroke, brain infections, and other neurological conditions. Referrals still steadily come into *our service. And those who have already suffered any of these, of course, still need on-going rehabilitation, care and support – even if they have also contracted Covid-19.*

April 16, 2020
The roads are so quiet that I arrive way too early for my liking at the hospital. I am for once spoilt for choice for parking. Now the time has arrived to enter the unknown. I have been asked to see a person who had recently sustained a brain injury, and subsequently contracted Covid-19, on the isolation ward. What will it be like? Is it as bad as the daily news suggests? Nothing could have prepared me for what I see next. The entrance to the hospital is locked, in broad daylight. Surely there is a mistake, hospitals are always open? Let me have a look around. A hastily scribbled note taped to the inside of the window next to the entrance to the hospital says, 'shout for attention' (I have a photograph of this). A receptionist lets me in and looks at me stunned. They walk me through silent corridors to the ward, where I am met by a nurse who will help me with what I have no idea yet how to do. Everything is new to me, showering, changing into blue scrubs (the nurse chooses a size for me after a quick cursory glance at me), then PPE, and then, they indicate I am 'good to go'. For the record, the scrubs that were confidently deemed to be 'your perfect size' were, shall we say, a tad too big for me... I have a photograph of them to prove that!
Once dressed in my way too loose blue outfit with matching plastic and a visor, now, finally, I step for the first time, into the isolation ward – essentially a 'ward within a ward'. It is a very visceral experience, unlike

anything else I have experienced in a hospital. It feels, no, it is, very hot inside. The PPE visor bathes the scene in a distorted soft focus, and there is a lot of coughing and calling for help. But there is nothing 'soft focus' in the world immediately outside of the visor. The air is stale and dry with fear. Outside the sun is shining brightly through a huge window, and into the ward. I do a bedside cognitive assessment and take a history from the person I had been asked to see. All the time, I am very aware of my own breathing, slowly in, slowly out. What is entering my lungs, I briefly wonder.

When I exit the isolation ward, I don't think I get the order of taking off all my PPE quite right. The nurse helps me and tells me to go and shower. The shower afterwards in the hospital changing room does nothing to wash off my feelings about what I had just witnessed. I wash myself several times. Outside the sun is shining brightly through the windscreen of my car as I drive back, wondering if I will get sick, and what that would mean. Of course, being human, there is no denying that I start to consider 'the odds' of losing. To name the demon, I briefly wonder if I would die if I got infected with Covid-19 in the ward today. It's difficult to comprehend and not something I can talk to someone about. In silence, just the soothing noise of the grey tarmac ribbon of the road slowly but progressively being reeled in under the red bonnet of my car, I notice that I am still breathing really slowly.

May 29, 2020
It's a long walk along the familiar passages to a ward I know well. But the passages seem alien today. Eerily quiet. I have not seen a soul yet, which is unusual.

Where is everybody? Even the dining room off the corridor is empty. Walking along the corridor, my footsteps echo as if I am engaging in some 'dark tourism' in a foreign country, to visit an abandoned building with a tragic past. I stop. Things have very much changed since I was last here. The ward entrance is closed. It is now a case of PPE-up before ringing the bell to be let in. Inside it is busy. Everyone is busy by a bed or walking towards a bay. Light is reflected off the visors clinical staff milling about are wearing. An army of light green plastic figures. It could be a scene from a 1960s science fiction space travel movie. Only thing is we are not in a movie, even though this could as well have been a new planet.

Several of the multi-disciplinary team members are new to this ward, seconded from other (non-neuro) departments of the Trust. They are very friendly and seem pleased to have me join them. I am asked to see one of the new patients, who has a memory problem. The real problem is that they cannot remember their password for their laptop, making it impossible for them to remain in touch with the outside world and their loved ones. It is very hard for me to figure out what underpins their memory problem. Compliments of my visor, I am looking at a strangely distorted person in front of me, and there are multiple voices speaking in the background din of people working around the neighbouring beds. But eventually, after trying to move the laptop across their visual field, I finally figure out that their memory problem is in fact a visual neglect common to a lesion in a certain area of the brain, commonly caused by a Stroke. It transpires both of us could not see the world as it should be, but for very different reasons.

June 3, 2020
I am back in the same (isolation) ward. The work tempo
is fast. From one room to the next. Then back to the
bays. In one of the side rooms, one of the patients asked
me if we are all going to die in here. I don't know the
answer but try to reassure them as best as I can, by
speaking from my heart, 'I cannot see any reason why
that would happen'. They seem to take some solace from
that. Me too. As a clinician-scientist, I cannot predict
the future. But I truthfully cannot envisage how all of
us in the ward at this moment, will die of Covid-19. As
I walk back to the parking area outside along the long,
empty hospital corridors; I reconsider my statement.
Yes, not <u>all</u> of us, but... Oof, I'm in the wrong part of
the car park! I was distracted and must have briefly for-
gotten where I parked.

June 10, 2020
Back in the red wards of one of the main hospitals today.
Increasingly, I am becoming aware of how difficult it is
for me to recognise colleagues I know from the past. We
are all masked figures with a range of emotions saying
what we don't say through our eyes when catching a
person's gaze. Sometimes a tiny bead of sweat on the
forehead, or red blotches in the neck confirms what the
eyes are silently saying. It's a tough place to be. A person
in a side room here in the red ward made me think. They
presented with profound suspiciousness about their
situation: why they were in this strange place and what
were these people around them doing? I assumed that
the presentation was the result of a recently acquired
brain injury (Stroke). But I could not help wondering –
if I were to be trapped in a ward in this strange new

world of Covid-19, would I not also become suspicious about what was actually happening? I feel deeply sorry for them, and the situation they find themselves in. I wish I could make it better.

June 17, 2020
One of the people I saw in an isolation ward earlier this month is now gravely ill with Covid-19. I have come to see them in a medical ward. They are so unwell that they can barely open their eyes to respond to my question. They are on constant observation by an agency worker – who started today and can tell me very little about my patient – how they have been, any changes? Staff sickness has started to take its toll on the NHS and there is increasing reliance on agency workers. The feeling of heat and the smell of stale air and illness is slowly choking me. I feel incredibly powerless and, at the same time, desperately sorry for the patient, fearing what might happen to them. It's not clear if science will be able to save them.

The relief when I get outside into the fresh air and sunshine, after finishing my attempt to assess the patient, is indescribable. It is like what I imagine a near drowning experience must feel like, making it to the surface and being able to breathe again. It must be unimaginably hard for hospital staff who work 12-hour non-stop shifts, and who don't have the luxury of going outside. Driving back to the unit along a road next to the ocean, I start to wonder about the patient I have just seen. They are so utterly alone in their struggle to breathe, to keep on hanging in there. Just a little crumpled, almost motionless, semi-curled-up bundle, floating in and out of who knows what. What will become of them? I stop my car. There is a small, no, very small with only six seats, chapel dating back to the time of a 6ᵗʰ century saint. The altar is over a well, the water of which were thought to have healing powers. As a clinician-scientist I don't have the right words but silently, on my own, in the dim light of the cool, quiet chapel ask that the patient would please be okay and survive.

June 24, 2020

Today I am working at a community hospital normally covered by one of my colleagues. We decided that colleagues with young children ideally should do remote (digital) working to protect them and their children. I perform a bedside cognitive assessment and decide, based on the patient's present cognitive function, that there isn't a robust reason why they cannot be discharged and go home, provided they are medically well enough. Driving back to my next stop – the red wards – I reflect that even through the haze and distortions of PPE and the emotions of the pandemic, neuropsychology still has something useful to offer patients and the multi-disciplinary team. The sooner patients can go home when able to and any required support is in place, the better. Home is almost always best, and even more so now.

June 25, 2020

I am at a local nursing home. I am reviewing the very first patient I saw back in April, who had a brain injury and Covid-19 at the time I first saw them (journal entry April 16, 2020). It's a mix of joy and relief to see that they did not succumb to the illness. They cannot remember seeing me at the time they were so unwell in the isolation ward. Given how ill they were, I am not entirely surprised by that. From a clinical perspective, it is striking to see how much less fatigued they are compared to April. It is an important learning point – some of the clinical features of Covid-19 can obscure or overlap with those of brain injury. There are, in fact, several factors to consider when assessing patients who have Covid-19: not only fatigue or poor concentration, but also psychological factors such as anxiety, the fact that everything takes longer, and the perceptual challenges posed to both parties by the clinician wearing PPE (Coetzer, 2020).

July 1, 2020
A day in the ward where I now go on a regular basis. We are learning more and more about Covid-19, including the fact that people (sadly not all) do recover from the illness. There is a strange solace in this realisation, or perhaps it is just that statistics and data can be frightening or reassuring. Just depends on which side of the numbers fence you find yourself on. At the end of the day, I check my emails. There is an email from a relative to cancel a home visit for later this week. I do the mathematics. I saw them a few days ago at home. The numbers indicate that to be ill now, they would definitely have already had the virus during my visit. It is the phase where a person already has Covid-19 but aren't yet displaying any symptoms. This is the time when whoever is in contact with them – clinician, friend, relative, shopkeeper – potentially unknowingly steps into the abyss of the unknown. A part of my work I tried not to think about, without much success. They are now critically ill in hospital, having suffered organ failure. I feel

a sense of fear for them, and their family and hope that they will be okay. I also hope that my PPE protected me in the no man's land of playing hide and seek with pre-symptomatic Covid-19, and that on this occasion I will be on the right side of the numbers. There's nothing else one can do. No amount of rumination can change things.

October 20, 2020
The hospital in-patient ward where I now go two days per week. It is an unusually short journal entry, simply mentioning that I saw five patients who had recently suffered an acquired brain injury, and that 'I hope I can sustain the pace'. Even my handwriting looks exhausted. It is exactly seven months since we left Africa on one of the last flights back to the UK. It feels like seven years ago though. When will it end?

(xii) Key Workers: Risk and Relationships

Although most of the population had to stay at home, either working virtually or on furlough, there was an essential group in society who needed to carry on going out to do their jobs with the NHS to provide essential health services and in other sectors to keep critical systems running. During the pandemic, these key workers faced a huge amount of uncertainty about the level of risk they were facing, often with inadequate PPE. There were serious and frightening implications of catching the virus when treatments were scarce and so many people were getting seriously ill and tragically dying. Those in the health service were very much 'on the front line', coming into direct contact with patients who had

Covid-19, and facing the challenge of coping with the practicalities of PPE. There were also innumerable other key workers providing critical services to keep our communities safe and functioning.

[Rudi]
As Sue very rightly points out, all around me, us, there were people who were performing high risk jobs, daily, and who were often taken for granted. Shopping felt more risky than everyday work in the hospital. Excluding the high-risk work in the isolation and red wards, the rest of my work in the hospital felt safer than going to a super-market. In the 'normal' hospital wards there was the constant use of PPE and controlling the environment, as well as first screening anyone you came in contact with clinically. In the supermarket there was no con-trol over how many times a bunch of bananas had been twirled around, examined, potentially coughed on, and inspected before being discarded as 'not quite right'. Before being bought by myself. Before being checked out by an unsuspecting cashier. These were the poor cashiers and other store staff who often had little in the way of PPE or barriers, who were being exposed to thousands of people every day – some of whom didn't wear a mask or consistently cleaned their hands. I felt very sorry for these and other 'hidden' essential workers who kept the UK daily living show on the road, without much thanks or praise for going way over the extra mile to keep us comfortable.

Many key workers also had families at home – partners, children, parents – and had to face the emotional and practical challenges of how to keep those they loved safe in the event of potentially being in close contact with other people who might have the virus. At this point, we knew so little about the virus, apart from that 'anyone could have it, and anyone could pass it on'. The invisible, asymptomatic aspects of Covid-19 made it very difficult to know for sure if someone might be a 'carrier' of the virus and inadvertently act as an unsuspecting conduit for transmission. There was also a lot of concern about how it might be transmitted, whether that was by touch or breathing, to the extent that many of us were rinsing off our shopping and putting parcels aside for a '3 day quarantine'.

My partner Mike was one of the Key Workers during the pandemic, working on critical national high voltage infrastructure (or as he put it 'someone has to keep the lights on'). As a senior electrical engineer he had to return to work, going out to site or in the shared office, and by the very nature of the job he often worked with other people. Whilst he did not knowingly come into contact with anyone with Covid-19, in the early stages of the pandemic we really did not know the level of potential risk. In the context of being told by the Prime Minister that most of us had to avoid ALL contact with other people, it seemed at the time to be very risky to be in proximity to anyone else at all.

From the very start after my accident, Mike had been my main 'support person', essential for helping me in the early days to manage even the basics of daily living. Over the next few years, he would continue to be the only person who saw much of what I was experiencing – the fatigue, the cognitive confusion, the shutdowns. My brain injury didn't just affect me, but also my relationship with my partner and often his life too, frequently restricting activities that we had previously enjoyed and dealing with the inevitable cognitive crashes when things got too much for my brain. It was a path we walked together, trying to learn and cope as we went on, and I will be forever grateful for this. Despite being inherently independent, and my determination to prove that I could do everything on my own, I was often reliant on his support, both practically and emotionally, as I tried to understand and manage my brain injury and its various challenges.

So when the pandemic hit and Mike was called back in to work, we were faced with a dilemma. For over ten years we had happily lived in separate houses, seeing each other frequently but maintaining our independence and autonomy. However, the government made it clear that we were only allowed to mix with our own 'household' and that couples who were currently living apart should either move in together or not see each other at all. Neither of those options would be right for me and Mike. Obviously the government advice really hadn't had the opportunity to consider the impacts this might have on someone with a brain injury and cognitive impairments, nor the impact these have on daily life and the challenge these impairments present to either living with someone or living apart! My brain injury meant that I needed a lot of 'quiet time', existing in silence for a large part of the day to reduce the impact of my difficulties with sensory overload and selective attention. Having another person permanently in the house, even one as understanding as my partner, would be too much for my brain as the sound of someone moving around and talking would be catastrophic when I needed a total absence of any stimuli. At the same time, the emotional and practical challenges of having a brain injury meant that his support was also critical to my ability to cope. So going it completely alone was not an option, even more so when faced with the changes to my functional routines like shopping which had been brought in as a result of the restrictions of the pandemic.

The most practical solution was to remain in separate houses and see each other when we could to provide support and social contact. Fortunately the lockdown regulations allowed people to provide care and help to a vulnerable person. Much as I disliked the label of 'vulnerable', I had to acknowledge that I needed some support to manage my brain injury. It was very much appreciated that Rudi, as my clinical neuropsychologist, was able to write an official NHS letter that named my partner as my support person. So for the first time ever Mike carried a letter in the car every time he came over to my house, an essential document to justify driving in the event of being stopped and questioned by the police.

The biggest challenge we both faced was about the relative risk of Mike being in contact with other people at work, and the decision about whether or not he was 'safe' to come over to see me. My house had rapidly become my sanctuary in the pandemic, and my front door was a secure gateway through which no-one else was allowed to pass. The constant need to question Mike about who he had seen, for how long, and how close they had been to each other felt so intrusive. We had never previously pried into each other's lives in such detail, respecting our right to live our lives independently. It started to make me increasingly anxious, the repeated worry about how much risk was involved, and the lack of autonomy in choosing that level of risk as it was up to Mike to make those decisions at work.

[Rudi]
From the moment we arrived back from our disastrous attempt to holiday in the sunshine of Africa, my friend and I knew we were inevitably going to face a problem. Unless you are comfortable playing a lottery with unknown odds, this was going to be a big problem, whichever way you look at it. My friend is a data scientist, she knows a thing or three about numbers, odds ratios, and significance. A small square foot living space plus one of the two occupants going into high-risk environments (hospitals) every day while the other is confined to full-time home-based working, is not a good formula, whichever way you try to make the numbers be more reassuring. You don't need a data scientist to figure that out. We had not been living together for very long when the pandemic arrived. It was bad timing, to say the least. It was impossible to move. For the foreseeable future, home was going to be here, or nowhere.

I often felt very guilty for exposing my friend to a potentially high level of risk even though we agreed that the situation we found ourselves trapped in was unfortunately just the way life turned out for us. There wasn't much to do other than meticulous use of PPE and handwashing, plus close monitoring of any suspicious symptoms such as a raised temperature. It also helped to quickly learn what were the differences between dehydration (common with wearing PPE throughout the day), exhaustion, or anxiety, as opposed to something suggesting an infection – which of course may or may not be early symptoms suggestive of Covid-19. Within days of the pandemic coughing was demoted from 'shame, are you okay, have some water' to 'what do you think you are doing, have you lost your mind, go away!' Later, the availability of lateral flow testing (LFT) and vaccination, made a big difference to being more able to protect others.

With time, developing routines proved helpful and emotionally reassuring. In a time of uncertainty, having something predictable provided the small daily anchors to bring calmness, a tiny dose of certainty, and mark the passing of time in what felt like an open-ended chapter. These routines included the decision on the second day after returning from Africa to do daily exercise, outside, no matter what the weather. No skipping of any days. No excuses were to be acceptable. Goals normally have an end point to measure success against, but open-ended goals are psychologically much harder to complete. However, somewhere along the marching on of time and the decision to record daily exercising this routine slowly morphed into a habit, which lives on to this day (at the time of writing, March 2025). Daily exercise outside in effect became its own story, divorced from the pandemic for a long time already now. An interesting study by Boere *et al.* (2023) *showed that while we already know exercise is good for us, exercising outside is particularly beneficial from a cognitive and brain well-being per-spective. In fact, a recent paper by* Zayatz *et al.* (2024) *found that regularly exercising outside during the pan-demic was associated with reduced stress levels.*

Another routine, or perhaps more of a 'ritual' was 'the daily scrubs washing mission'. In the early days, when I asked a colleague (one of the four secondees mentioned earlier) about this conundrum, they confidently said to me that they opened all hospital doors by pushing with their torso or hips against the door, so that their hands never touched any surfaces and were super clean. No need to wear gloves the whole day. When I tongue in cheek then asked how they took off their scrubs at the end of the day, there was a much longer pause than after my first question! At home, the ritual was scrubs off first, into the machine, select higher temperature setting, powder in, press start, hands next, hope for the best. Later in the pandemic clinical staff had to change on the ward before going home. There were lots of other things like 'work' trainers, and 'home' trainers (if you are going to stand for long periods, shoes have to be comfortable), timing of shopping, exercising at night when it is quiet, and watching too much Netflix over weekends in an attempt to escape any thoughts or reminders of what was outside the apartment and which had to be faced again from Monday. And of course, alcohol. You can never have too much alcohol hand sanitising gel in the house, should the supermarkets run out of soap!

It was not a Monday, but instead a Tuesday (journal entry, July 21, 2020) when after a day in the hospital I went back after work to see the patient (see above, journal entry, July 1, 2020) who had been admitted to hospital critically ill with Covid-19 after my community home visit. Their relative contacted me earlier to say that they were discharged from hospital and at home, and that they'd like to see me for the cancelled review now. As I PPE up outside the house, I notice in the afternoon light a beautiful colourful banner made by their children, to celebrate the fact that their parent survived

Covid-19. It hangs defiantly above a window, outside the house. Inside, feeling like I am in a dream seeing them sit right in front of me, alive, I get on with things and do the clinical review. From a neuropsychological perspective there has been no change in cognition, mood, or behaviour. Their level of fatigue though is striking but expected after being gravely ill with Covid-19. They are very grateful that I came out to review them. Outside, from the trapped summer warmth in my car, I look at the banner again and am suddenly overwhelmed by very strong emotions. It's time to go but I must first wait a bit to make sure I can properly see before I reverse out of the driveway towards a busy road where life goes on.

A large-scale study (Topriceanu et al., 2021) based on the UK's longitudinal surveys into the impact of the first national lockdown in 2020 on Key Workers found that there was a mixed picture of positive and negative effects. It found that, as expected, being a key worker was associated with an increased likelihood of being infected with Covid-19. However, interestingly at the time of the first lockdown, being a key worker was not associated with more psychological distress, although the mental health impacts of the pandemic became much more apparent later on. Of significant note, there was an increase in their conflict with people around them. Understanding the mix of impacts reflects some of my experience of having a partner who was a Key Worker during the pandemic, even for people without a brain injury.

As many of the key workers were more exposed to COVID-19 than the rest of the population during lockdown, their infection rates were higher ... Key workers tended to experience more conflict with the people around them, some of which might have been augmented by relatives' fear of getting infected, or key workers' worries over bringing the virus home to their loved ones.

(Topriceanu et al., 2021)

Brain injury changes people's relationships with their partners and families. It impacts significantly on both the person with the brain injury and their partner, altering both their lives in similar and different ways. It can have both negative and positive effects, and these change over time as well.

For me, it altered the relative balance between us, from two equally independent individuals to an increasing shift towards a feeling of dependency. This was significantly exacerbated by the pandemic, and the impact of my partner going out to work whilst I stayed at home. Whilst he faced potential risks to his health from the virus, he could make those choices and decisions for himself. He also gained the psychological benefits of going out, seeing people, and having a sense of purpose and meaningful activity. In staying at home I very much appreciated that this kept me safe from the virus, but simultaneously, without me particularly realising it at the time, it started to significantly change my mental health with rising anxiety and stress levels. It was increasingly difficult for both of us and put a further strain on our relationship in addition to the challenges of adjusting to my brain injury.

As the pandemic continued, the stresses and strains for all of us started to rise. The risk from the virus started to affect our health not only as a potentially fatal respiratory disease, but also our wider health as the effects of exhaustion, grief, isolation and uncertainty began to kick in.

References

Arnold, C. (2018). *Pandemic 1918*. Michael O'Mara Books.

Beal, E., Pelser, C., & Coates, P. (2023). Lockdown life–experiences of partners of individuals with an acquired brain injury during the COVID-19 pandemic: A qualitative study. *Brain Impairment, 24*, 260–273. https://doi.org/10.1017/BrImp.2023.7

Boere, K., Lloyd, K., Binsted, G., & Krigolson, O. E. (2023). Exercising is good for the brain but exercising outside is potentially better. *Scientific Reports, 13*(1), 1–8.

Burton, A. E., & Elliott, J. M. (2023). A mixed methods exploration of a pilot photo-reflection intervention for enhancing coping and well-being during COVID-19. *The Arts in Psychotherapy, 82*, 101990. https://doi.org/10.1016/j.aip.2022.101990

Byrne, C., Salas, C. E., Coetzer, R., & Ramsey, R. (2022). Understanding loneliness in brain injury: Linking the reaffiliation motive model of loneliness with a model of executive impairment. *Frontiers in Integrative Neuroscience, 16*, 883746. https://doi.org/10.3389/fnint.2022.883746

Coetzer, R. (2020). First impressions of performing bedside cognitive assessment of COVID-19 inpatients. *Journal of the American Geriatrics Society, 68*(7), 1389–1390. https://doi.org/10.1111/jgs.16561

Coetzer, R. (2015). A picture tells a lifetime of words: Photography, psychotherapy, and brain injury rehabilitation. *Neuro-Disability and Psychotherapy, 3*(1), 1–10.

George, A. J., Mathew, D. E., Lazarus, E., Chichra, A., Singh, B., & Gaikwad, P. (2021, August 19). Effectiveness of self-portraits used over personal protective equipment during the COVID-19 pandemic among patients and healthcare workers. *British Journal of Surgery, 108*(8), e270–e271. doi: https://doi.org/10.1093/bjs/znab138

Headway. (2020). *The impact of lockdown on brain injury survivors and their families.* www.headway.org.uk/media/8564/the-impact-of-lockdown-on-brain-injury-survivors-and-their-families.pdf

Howlett, J. R., Nelson, L. D., & Stein, M. B. (2022). Mental health consequences of traumatic brain injury. *Biological Psychiatry, 91*(5), 413–420.

Kaplan, R., & Kaplan, S. (1989). *The experience of nature: A psychological perspective.* Cambridge University Press.

Lassaletta, A. (2020). *The invisible brain injury.* Routledge.

Levy, C. E., Uomoto, J. M., Betts, D. J., & Hoenig, H. (2025). Creative arts therapies in rehabilitation. *Archives of Physical Medicine and Rehabilitation, 106*(1), 153–157. https://doi.org/10.1016/j.apmr.2024.07.008

Lorenz, L. S. (2012). Brain injury survivors: Narratives of rehabilitation and healing. *Visual Studies, 27*(2), 217–218.

Manthorpe, J., Iliffe, S., Gillen, P., Moriarty, J., Mallett, J., Schroder, H., Currie, D., Ravalier, J., & McFadden, P. (2022). Clapping for carers in the Covid-19 crisis: Carers' reflections in a UK survey. *Health & Social Care in the Community, 30*(4), 1442–1449. https://doi.org/10.1111/hsc.13474

Mantovani, E., Zucchella, C., Bottiroli, S., Federico, A., Giugno, R., Sandrini, G., Chiamulera, C., & Tamburin, S. (2020). Telemedicine and virtual reality for cognitive rehabilitation: A roadmap for the COVID-19 pandemic. *Frontiers in Neurology, 11*, 926. https://doi.org/10.3389/fneur.2020.00926

May, T., Aughterson, H., Fancourt, D., & Burton, A. (2021). 'Stressed, uncomfortable, vulnerable, neglected': A qualitative study of the psychological and social impact of the COVID-19 pandemic on UK frontline keyworkers. *BMJ Open*, 11(11), e050945.

McDonnell, A. S., & Strayer, D. L. (2024). Immersion in nature enhances neural indices of executive attention. *Science Reports*, *14*, 1845. https://doi.org/10.1038/s41598-024-52205-1

Morrow, E. L., Patel, N. N., & Duff, M. C. (2021). Disability and the COVID-19 pandemic: A survey of individuals with traumatic brain injury. *Archives of Physical Medicine and Rehabilitation*, *102*(6), 1075–1083.

Ohly, H., White, M. P., Wheeler, B. W., Bethel, A., Ukoumunne, O. C., Nikolaou, V., & Garside, R. (2016). Attention restoration theory: A systematic review of the attention restoration potential of exposure to natural environments. *Journal of Toxicology and Environmental Health. Part B, Critical Reviews*, *19*(7), 305–343. https://doi.org/10.1080/10937404.2016.1196155

Rice, W. L., Mateer, T. J., Reigner, N., Newman, P., Lawhon, B., & Taff, B. D. (2020). Changes in recreational behaviors of outdoor enthusiasts during the COVID-19 pandemic: Analysis across urban and rural communities. *Journal of Urban Ecology*, *6*(1), juaa020. https://doi.org/10.1093/jue/juaa020

Salas, C. E., Casassus, M., Rowlands, L., Pimm, S., & Flanagan, D. A. J. (2016). "Relating through sameness": A qualitative study of friendship and social isolation in chronic traumatic brain injury. *Neuropsychological Rehabilitation*, *28*(7), 1161–1178. https://doi.org/10.1080/09602011.2016.1247730

Solomon, Z., Mikulincer, M., Ohry, A., & Ginzburg, K. (2021). Prior trauma, PTSD long-term trajectories, and risk for PTSD during the COVID-19 pandemic: A 29-year longitudinal study. *Journal of Psychiatric Research, 141,* 140–145.

Stockwell, S., Trott, M., Tully, M., Shin, J., Barnett, Y., Butler, L., ... & Smith, L. (2021). Changes in physical activity and sedentary behaviours from before to during the COVID-19 pandemic lockdown: A systematic review. *BMJ Open Sport & Exercise Medicine, 7,* e000960.

Taleb, S., Vahedian-Azimi, A., Karimi, L., Salim, S., Mohammad, F., Samhadaneh, D., ... & Ait Hssain, A. (2024). Evaluation of psychological distress, burnout and structural empowerment status of healthcare workers during the out-break of coronavirus disease (COVID-19): A cross-sectional questionnaire-based study. *BMC Psychiatry, 24,* 61.

Topriceanu, C. C., Wong, A., Moon, J. C., Hughes, A. D., Chaturvedi, N., Conti, G., ... & Captur, G. (2021). Impact of lockdown on key workers: Findings from the COVID-19 survey in four UK national longitudinal studies. *Journal of Epidemiology and Community Health, 75,* 1–8. https://doi.org/10.1136/jech-2020-215889

Tyerman, A., Buckle, C., King, N., & Melville, J. (2021). Remote contact during Covid-19 lockdown: Feedback from people with brain injury. *Neuropsychologist, 11,* 4.

Van Praag, D. L. G., Cnossen, M. C., Polinder, S., Wilson, L., & Maas, A. I. R. (2019). Post-traumatic stress dis-order after civilian traumatic brain injury: A systematic review and meta-analysis of prevalence rates. *Journal of Neurotrauma,* 36(23), 3220–3232. https://doi.org/10.1089/neu.2018.5759

Venter, Z. S., Barton, D. N., Gundersen, V., Figari, H., & Nowell, M. S. (2021). Back to nature: Norwegians sustain increased recreational use of urban green space months after the COVID-19 outbreak. *Landscape and Urban Planning, 214,* 104175.

Vibholm, A. P., Christensen, J. R., & Pallesen, H. (2020). Nature-based rehabilitation for adults with acquired brain injury: A scoping review. *International Journal of Environmental Health Research, 30*(6), 661–676. https://doi.org/10.1080/09603123.2019.1620183

Wilson, L., Horton, L., Kunzmann, K., Sahakian, B. J., Newcombe, V. F., Stamatakis, E. A., ... & Menon, D. (2021). Understanding the relationship between cognitive performance and function in daily life after traumatic brain injury. *Journal of Neurology, Neurosurgery & Psychiatry, 92*, 407–417.

Wong, M. M. Y., Seliman, M., Loh, E., Mehta, S., & Wolfe, D. L. (2022). Experiences of Individuals Living with Spinal Cord Injuries (SCI) and Acquired Brain Injuries (ABI) during the COVID-19 Pandemic. *Disabilities, 2*(4), 750–763. https://doi.org/10.3390/disabilities2040052

Yeo, T. J. (2020). Sport and exercise during and beyond the COVID-19 pandemic. *European Journal of Preventive Cardiology, 27*(12), 1239–1241. https://doi.org/10.1177/2047487320933260

Zayatz, C., Kruger, J., Drozdowsky, J., & Anzman-Frasca, S. (2024). Associations between daily activities, stress, and sleep among adults during the COVID-19 pandemic. *American Journal of Lifestyle Medicine, 18*(3), 313–322.

Chapter 4

More Change
Will it Ever End?

Sue Williams and Rudi Coetzer

(i) Lockdown Ends

As the pandemic progressed into the summer of 2020, the first strict lockdown eased, and the UK began a process of changing rules and regulations regarding social mixing and travel. In June, the instructions were eased a bit more to permit activities in a wider area, although people in Wales still had to 'stay local', which was defined as within five miles. Importantly, people were allowed to mix in groups of six. By July, travel restrictions were lifted and 'extended households' were permitted. Although people were still encouraged to limit themselves to small groups of six, the regulations allowed for larger gatherings of up to 30 (for example, for a wedding). To make this more confusing, the rules were often different in England compared to Wales. This created several challenges: people from places without restrictions visiting other areas where residents were still limiting contact; differences between what family and friends in England and Wales were allowed to do and who was allowed to meet up at certain times; and increasingly fractious debate about what was 'safe'.

The changing rules and regulations, along with how they varied across regions and timescales, presented me

DOI: 10.4324/9781003509134-7

with a significant cognitive challenge. Like many people with a brain injury, I had learnt early on that any change was much harder to cope with than before my brain injury, even with the smallest of things. Trying to keep as much as possible in my life the same helped me by reducing the need to consider and evaluate options and make decisions, which therefore meant that I could use my limited cognitive capacity for other things. So before the pandemic, I had to just go to the same supermarket, buy the same products, walk the same paths and try to keep things in the same place. In effect, I tried to 'auto-pilot' as much as possible in my life. As someone who had previously lived life in a somewhat 'ad-hoc' way, perfectly capable of adjusting in a dynamic way in response to any change, I had been surprised by my new preference for routine after my brain injury. However, I now found it so much easier to do things in the same way. Disruption to my routines would leave me feeling like the proverbial 'bear with a sore head', with frustration often adding to the cognitive demands of adjusting to different situations and the consequential increase in neurological fatigue. 'Why can't they just leave things the same?' I would often mutter to myself when I found things had changed.

> It's good for people with brain injury to stick to routines in familiar surroundings where they can predict what is going to happen and what resources they have. This way, they can dedicate attention to other tasks, and don't need to improvise their performance while they're on the go. Improvising is highly demanding for our brain!
>
> (Bilbao and Diaz, 2008, quoted in Lassaletta, 2020)

The Covid-19 lockdown presented a huge change, and my routines went out the window, so I had to do things differently. As I've discussed, even the simple difference of having to change my food shopping from my 'normal supermarket' to buying what I could online using various supermarkets, caused me to struggle with the extra cognitive demands that this placed on my brain. I was not alone in this, and many people with a brain injury also struggled with the disruption to their daily routines. Nearly 70% of the respondents to a national survey of brain injury survivors stated that changes to their routine had disrupted their daily life (Headway, 2020).

Despite this, during the first lockdown, I did eventually settle down into a new simple routine as described in the previous chapters, with local walks and a few regular online activities. Even online food shopping became a bit easier as it became more familiar and I no longer had to shop for others as they set up their own accounts and local support. I had become more used to my rehab sessions on the phone with Rudi, and talking remotely felt much more comfortable. For several months, the rules and regulations had stayed the same and applied equally to everyone, regardless of where we lived or how many cases there were in our area. After working through some of my initial fears and flashbacks triggered by the risk of the virus, I felt relatively safe. Although often lonely, I had the support of my partner and online contact with my family and friends, which helped to mitigate the isolation. For my brain, this had become my 'new normal' and it no longer presented such a psychological and cognitive strain.

So when the regulations changed in July 2020, we all had to adjust to a new way of doing things again. Similar to the first lockdown, this change presented some benefits and challenges when we were all eventually released from many of the significant restrictions which had been in place for so long. What would this new way of living mean for my brain? How would this 'opening up' affect my mental health? What did it mean for Rudi working within the NHS?

[Rudi]
Sue very eloquently in the text above describes how, during the first lockdown, we eventually settled into very predictable routines and how these were protective to us. These routines anchored life and provided the psychological scaffolding required to, without respite, just 'work, go home, eat, exercise outside, sleep, repeat'. Looking back now at photos from summer 2020, there are endless photos of landscapes or scenes, but as regards people, only ever my friend and I. Mostly of us hiking trails in Snowdonia, which begin very near where we lived. These photos are very colourful and she's almost always smiling in them. Me too, but there are quite a few where I am not and it's difficult to gauge from the photo what I might be feeling or thinking. Then in October, for the first time, there are four of us outside hiking! The weather had turned and although we are all smiling for the camera, it is clear that the cold of early winter had started to take hold.

(ii) Reconnecting

Although I had been fortunate to have regular online contact with friends and family and joined in with various virtual activities, this was ultimately not a complete substitute for seeing people in person. It seems strange nowadays, but back then the decision to meet up with someone seemed like a massive event. It was a big step, but finally I met up for a walk with a very close friend again.

Sue's Journal July 18, 2020
Wow, I finally met up with J again! It feels like forever since I've seen her. I mean, we've messaged online, but it's not the same. To be able to smile, see each other, chat and laugh about so many things. It was like 'look you've still got legs and a bum' – I haven't been able to see anything more than your top half on a screen for so long! My heart is singing with the joy of seeing her again. But I was quite anxious too. It's not easy to stay two metres apart, even outdoors, the path isn't always that wide. I hope we didn't get too close. I trust J completely, but it still feels quite risky for both of us. We only met up for an hour and went for a little walk, but I'm exhausted now.

I don't think I was prepared for the effect of adjusting to seeing people in person again after being unable to have that type of contact for so long, nor the complex emotions that this would bring. The impact isolation had had on our social skills has been well documented, and I certainly felt very stilted and rusty. For someone who had previously been able to 'talk the hind leg off a donkey', it was strange to not feel my words flow so easily.

However, for me the challenge of talking was not just due to the effect of a lack of in-person social engagement during the lockdown. Since the start of my brain injury, I had been having difficulties with communication. As described in previous chapters, to begin with, after my accident, I was literally unable to talk. My badly broken jaw, displaced teeth, facial injuries and torn trachea meant that I could not open my mouth or move my jaw. So initially, my intermittent attempts at communication were reliant on short written notes as I could not speak at all. As I healed, I slowly began to mumble, although this continued to be a painful experience. My injuries had caused significant nerve damage in my lower face, some of which remains to this day. For the first few years, my lower face felt very stiff and lacked sensitivity, in the same way as the effects of a dental anaesthetic. So the physical processes of being able to speak was very challenging, and I continued to feel self-conscious about this, worried about how I was sounding and constantly feeling the sensation of 'dribbling' out the side of my mouth even though this wasn't happening.

However, it was the difficulties I experienced within my brain that caused me the greatest challenge with communication. Initially, my mental 'filing cabinet' of words was completely disordered and I frequently could not think of the right word for what I wanted to say. I seemed to no longer have an accurate awareness of my 'tone of voice'. It wasn't just an issue of being able to say words, but also to ensure that I conveyed the emotions in the same way. I was concerned that I was sounding angry or terse when I wanted to sound relaxed and friendly, but my ability to perceive my own intonation seemed to have disappeared. As time went on, I realised that I had some difficulties that were not going to go away.

Most significant was the cognitive process of speaking: the ability to think of the right word, find it in my head, capture it within the context of a sentence, keep hold of it and then manage to speak it out loud. Often, I had what I referred to as my 'tornado brain', where my words would be caught in a spiralling, out-of-control twister, swirling at speed in my head. I could 'feel' the words in my brain, but I could not capture them. They became like a pile of autumn leaves blown upwards in the wind, with me running round trying to grasp the single one that I needed to say. Exhausted by these attempts I would cease and slowly the cognitive whirlwind would drop. Like leaves, my words would slowly drift back down and settle in my brain again. But now they would be in complete disarray, landing in any which way, and I would lack the cognitive capacity and capability to search through them to find what I wanted to say.

Trying to explain this cognitive difficulty is almost impossible within the context of a normal conversation. Especially as, at the point when it is at its worst, I struggle to even say a simple single word like 'yes' or 'no'. Often in these situations, the early warning signals are when I start to stumble over my words, repeatedly saying 'um' as a cognitive stutter. If I try to persevere, I will become completely unable to speak. Although I can usually still hear what is being said near to me, I am unable to reply or respond verbally. It is a challenge that I still face to this day, although I have tried to manage it better by slowing down and taking a communication break.

Many of the impairments that I have described previously, such as my difficulties with attention, working memory and executive functions, combine to have an adverse effect on my ability to communicate verbally or to read. I have now learned that I have a Cognitive Communication Disorder, and like many of my problems, it is made worse by my neurological fatigue.

> Cognitive communication disorders (CCDs) are common in individuals with brain injury and may place a high burden on individuals and their family. The term CCD ... refers to communication dysfunction resulting from underlying deficits in one or more cognitive functions, such as attention, orientation, memory, information processing, reasoning, executive functions or social cognition.
>
> (Verhoeks, 2024)

I have great difficulties having a conversation in areas with competing stimuli due to attention issues, whilst my limited working memory makes it challenging to read a book (I often 'forget' the preceding sentence so end up reading the same paragraph over and over again), and I can have no recall of some things which I have heard or read. Writing this book has presented a real challenge in terms of my communication difficulties, as reading and reviewing what I have written can be very confusing and I often worry that I have written exactly the same thing several times. Equally, I can miss out words without realising it, or can put my letters the wrong way round in a way that I cannot see. I am therefore grateful for the help that I have had with proof-reading this book in draft form!

[Rudi]
Difficulties with social communication after TBI are very common, but often unrecognised. As Sue points out, several factors (including cognition, fatigue and anxiety) all conspire to make talking much harder than before and, especially so, in social situations. One way to explain this is to imagine that you are bilingual, or trilingual, but do not have complete mastery of the new languages you are still learning. Now imagine explaining something complex to another person, or being in a group where all of them are first language speakers of your second or third language. It's a new group and you are a bit apprehensive about getting to know them. Maybe that's the reason you did not sleep so well last night, now you are tired too. You struggle to keep track of what everyone is saying, your replies become slower and more effortful. 'They must think I am...' thoughts start to enter your mind. That doesn't help the anxiety, which in turn makes you more anxious. You get the picture of how it may feel for someone who has sustained a TBI. Now add a pandemic to the situation...

Like many aspects of my brain injury, my communication difficulties fluctuate. So at times, I can talk on the same level as everyone else. Although, my concern about my limited cognitive communication capacity means that I try to get what I want to say out as soon as possible in case it all goes awry in my brain. Unfortunately, this often means that when I am feeling cognitively capable of having a discussion, I talk 'a mile a minute' and I am aware that this can sometimes leave little space for other people to get a word in edgeways. However, this isn't due to a lack of interest in what others have to say; rather, I am always mindful of the extra effort that this takes out of my brain. I hide this from other people as much as I can, only 'having a chat' when I feel well rested and limiting the duration to ensure that I can retreat to somewhere quiet before it gets too much. On occasions, I have been caught out and ended up in difficult situations in public due to my inability to communicate. This has resulted in the police being called, or concern from ambulance paramedics, and my partner is usually essential in these situations as he can explain to others that my inability to speak is a 'brain issue' and will resolve if I am left alone to recover in silence. I now carry a Headway 'Brain Injury ID Card' with me when I go out, which explains to the police, paramedics or other people that I have communication difficulties.

As with many things, my cognitive communication disorder is made worse by stress and by lack of practice. So inevitably, the Covid-19 lockdown, with its limitations on in-person engagement, made it even harder for me to manage the communication difficulties that I have as a result of my brain injury. When we were allowed out to meet up with people in person again, I found that my ability to talk now felt so much more stilted, and 'chatting' was exhausting for me. I was in effect 'out of practice' and anxious, so this compounded my cognitive communication difficulties. I suspect that it wasn't that noticeable to my friends (or they were too polite to mention it), but I felt so self-conscious and constantly worried that I was going to start 'um-ing' and then shut down completely.

Whilst there are numerous self-reports that the lock-down caused social and communication difficulties for many people, as we began to emerge from lockdown, there was little mention of how this made things extra challenging for people like me with a pre-existing speech and language disorder. However, a report by the Royal College of Speech and Language Therapists (RCSLT) in the UK noted that the pandemic had resulted in an increased demand for their specialist services. Although some of this was due to the backlog that accrued during lockdown, the survey also noted:

> Another very commonly identified factor was "An increase in individuals requiring speech and language therapy due to deterioration/exacerbation of needs during lockdown."
>
> (RCSLT, 2022)

Despite my challenges with communication, it still felt incredible to meet up with people again. Unlike the period before the pandemic, when I had been alone in my lack of social contact, now we were all emerging from our individual boats in a sea of social isolation. Amongst my small group of close friends, we were all very cautious and carried some anxiety about what was 'safe' to do when we met up again. So we started what became known as our 'walk and talk' meets. Instead of a café, like many people, we now met up outdoors with a thermos and our sandwiches. For me, this had a double benefit. Firstly, it significantly reduced the risk of catching Covid-19 due to the fresh air, which in turn mitigated my anxiety. Secondly, as we were in a much quieter place, especially up in the mountains or on a deserted beach, my brain did not struggle with the attention and communication difficulties that I had previously experienced when trying to meet up with friends in a café before the pandemic.

I soon came to value these 'walk and talks' with my partner and a couple of close friends more than anything else. The overall quality of my social interactions improved no end compared to a life lived solely online, and my sense of isolation reduced significantly. Although different from my pre-brain-injury life, when I used to throw myself into social occasions with groups of colleagues and friends without the slightest issue, these one-to-one meet-ups led to an increased depth and quality of friendship than those before. With my small group of close friends, I developed meaningful and deep connections that I valued so much and still do so today.

The benefit of nature, which I have previously discussed, during the first pandemic lockdown was enhanced by my 'walk and talks' and the effect these had on my mental health. I found that walking side-by-side was less confrontational than being online and directly 'in your face' on a computer screen. This allowed more personal things to be discussed without being overly worried about the other person's immediate reactions. The movement of walking in itself, with its regular rhythm and active cardio-vascular processes, helped reduce my stress levels through this moderate physical activity.

Many others found a similar benefit from being able to go for a walk with a friend, or on their own, in green and natural spaces. Especially for people living in urban areas, with limited parks, the easing of lockdown meant that they could travel further to enjoy visits to the mountains and beaches across the UK. This presented a double-edged sword. On the one hand, it was extremely beneficial for so many people to be able to escape to the countryside. On the other hand, popular areas such as national parks and beaches soon had so many visitors that it presented real challenges for local communities. A comprehensive report on the impact of the pandemic on outdoor recreation and nature in the UK found that there were significant health and well-being benefits, but the 'reopening' of society caused a 're-bound effect' on visitor numbers with consequences for wildlife, land managers and local people:

> As lockdown restrictions were eased and places began to open up, increases in visitor numbers resulted in a range of problems for visitor experience and for site impact. These included overflowing litter, fly-tipping, deposits of human waste and a lack of public toilet facilities. A fear of overcrowding and inability to maintain safe social distances was exacerbated in some places by narrow pathways.
>
> (Armstrong et al., 2021)

As I live in a popular tourist area, the increase in visitors as lockdown restrictions eased caused a significant change, especially if compared to the previous months of the pandemic. Suddenly, all of my 'brain benefits' from lockdown, such as silence, a slower pace of life and a lack of nearby people, changed in my local area. Much as I appreciated the need for other people from urban areas to enjoy the opportunity to visit my local hills and the beach, it was far too much for me. There were too many people, it was too noisy, and it did not feel at all 'safe' to me. Consequently, my brain returned to being constantly overloaded and, even worse than before the pandemic, this was compounded by my significant increase in stress and anxiety about the transmission of the virus from so many people in close proximity.

So, despite the benefits of the easing of lockdown and the value of seeing a couple of close friends in person again, for me, the change in the regulations made my life harder. Fear, stress and anxiety, combined with neurological difficulties and fatigue to make my life increasingly distressing. This became the start of the hardest period of the pandemic for me. At times, I did not think I would make it through and wondered if this would ever end.

(iii) Fear and Threat

As lockdown eased, rather than feeling happier, my stress levels started to increase exponentially. The unholy trinity of brain injury, Covid-19 and trauma combined in ways that I did not expect. I was aware that my increasingly distressing emotions had a grounding in facts: the virus was a very real health threat, my brain injury affected my cognitive functions, and my traumatic experience had a significant visceral memory. However, the extent and magnitude of my psychological and behavioural response went beyond what might have been considered reasonable by many people, even myself; although I did not perceive it in that way at the time. In particular, what I did not yet understand was the impact that my brain injury had on regulating my emotions, especially those relating to stress and anxiety.

To begin with, I tried to subdue my anxiety and join in the increasing number of people who were feeling positive about the re-opening of society in albeit limited ways. Like the majority of us, I had spent the previous five months having 'DIY haircuts', standing in front of the bathroom mirror with my scissors, attempting to cut a straight line across my fringe so I could at least see! So when my local hairdresser said she was re-opening for limited individual appointments at her small salon, I booked a haircut. By now, the use of face masks had become increasingly recognised as an important measure to reduce the transmission of the virus, especially indoors. This would be my first foray into wearing a mask and meeting another person indoors since the start of the pandemic. Although my anxiety was bubbling away, I was certain I could manage this. After buying a simple DIY style mask online, when it arrived, I thought I'd just try it on to check if it would fit and to work out how I could attach it around my ears and still allow my hair to get cut.

Sue's Journal July 20, 2020

Mask! I'm still shaking as I write this. I picked up the mask without thinking much about it, I just wanted to check it would fit. I held it to my face, tightened the straps ... and I can't breathe ... I'm gasping, fighting, struggling for breath ... my fingers are scrabbling, scratching my face ... get it off, get it off ... I can't breathe ... all I can smell and taste is blood.

I'm back in time and place to my accident, on the road, in agony, choking on my blood, fighting the oxygen mask that the paramedics are trying to put on my face, convinced that they don't know that I can't breathe, that I'm drowning in blood and they don't understand that putting the oxygen mask on will kill me.

I got the DIY face mask off; it must have only been seconds, but it felt like eternity. A wave of nausea overcame me, and I only just made it to the bathroom before being sick. I'm shaking and sweating, my heart is racing. I crawled into bed and called Mum. Talking and crying on the phone. I feel so scared. Where did all this come from? What is happening to me?

Whilst it was obvious with hindsight that wearing a mask was another unexpected trigger for my post-traumatic flashbacks, that knowledge didn't really help with the day-to-day reality of managing during the pandemic. I tried several times to put the mask on again, but the shakes and fear would start before I'd even got it on my face. I felt so ashamed and guilty that I wasn't able to wear a face mask, even for a short time, especially as I was aware of how hard it was for health and care staff who had to try to cope with wearing masks and often full PPE for hours at a time, day after day. There was a small minority of the population who were vocal in being 'anti-mask' and I dreaded being associated with them as it wasn't that I didn't want to wear a mask, but rather that it provoked such terror that I struggled to even get it near to my face. However, to me it was really important to be responsible and wear a mask, so I persisted over and over again. I started off with a 'buff'

style face covering, slowly trying to subdue the flashbacks and become able to wear a face mask to protect
other people, no matter how long it took. It would be a
long time before I could manage this without fear, and it
was a lot easier to withdraw from seeing people indoors
instead, no matter how much I would have liked to meet
up with family and friends.

[Rudi]

*At work, everyone wore a mask. After work, many did
too, but not everyone. I was okay with that, and by now
understood that social distancing and not touching your
face, ever, were very effective behavioural precautions
we could take, plus washing hands, in the correct way,
regularly. If there was an alternative to alcohol – soap
and hot water was better, killing or getting rid of a wider
range of bugs if done properly. Masks were uncomfortable. Not initially, but by the afternoon, I always noticed
that despite drinking, I felt dehydrated. They also progressively, as the day wore on, became hotter and hotter.
The other thing was that by midday, the elastic of the
mask secured around your ears started to hurt. More
and more. However, as you adjusted the elastic, the area
behind your ears became progressively more sensitive.
And if you wore glasses, oh dear, the steaming up was
not great. Add the rest of the PPE and you had a perfect recipe for discomfort – though a necessary one for
health professionals, to protect those around us as well
as ourselves.*

*There were more protective masks available to
those of us who worked in high-risk areas. These were
Filtering Face Piece (FFP) masks, and you had to first
undergo Fit Testing before being cleared to use these.*

My date came and I shaved the previous night in antici-
pation of my test later the next day. The ward was busy
that morning, and I arrived a bit later in the afternoon
than anticipated. Unfortunately, I fell at the first hurdle
and failed the test. By this time in the day, my stub-
ble had decided to show and enjoy the sunshine. No
fit, no mask. After a few months working in high-risk
environments, I was called to attend an antibody test in
a field hospital. Pre-Covid-19, the 'field hospital' was
a theatre. Seeing a 'hospital' inside the place where I
used to watch shows was a bit confusing to process. A
very friendly nurse took my blood and that was that. In
and out in under five minutes. And the test? Well, I sort
of failed this one too. It transpired I had no antibodies,
which was interpreted as no immunity or defence
against Covid-19. This of course, was not an exact sci-
ence, and in any case, all became redundant once the
vaccines were developed months later. But for now, it
was back to the wards.

Unfortunately, I began to learn the hard way that trying
to suppress and control my heightened emotions in my
conscious mind meant that the fear would leak out at
night and take over my unconscious brain. I had struggled at times with sleep difficulties and nightmares after
my accident, but now this started to rise to an uncontrollable level. Over the summer and autumn of 2020,
as the weeks and months progressed with the easing
of lockdown and the emergence of people back to a
slightly more 'normal' life, my stress levels and consequent anxiety increased as more people began to visit
and socialise. To my mind, the threat of Covid-19 hadn't
disappeared; rather, it had only reduced in terms of the

number of cases. This meant that it was still 'out there' – invisible, sometimes asymptomatic and potentially carried by anyone. My fear fed off the daily updates of the cases of Covid-19, and although these were declining, it was obvious that the virus was not going to disappear completely.

Sue's Journal August 15, 2020

Fear has become my predominant emotion. Not just a bit anxious, not only a degree of stress, but a level of fear that feels like an explosive fire raging through me, uncontrollable and unstoppable. Heart racing, nausea rising, shaking and trembling … and yet often there was nothing physically there that was actually going to harm me. The fear has now spread from the dark hours of the night when it would catch me unawares, to the light of day as it grows more powerful and I become unable to manage it. It's like an uncontrollable ferocious beast, a fire-breathing dragon that will roar into life at the slightest provocation. Anything that feels like a perceived threat can provoke this response. I feel like I'm existing on a knife-edge, with a hairline trigger that will react to so many things. I'm scared of my own emotions now, how they take over like an out-of-control wildfire. I wish I could stop it; I am absolutely exhausted. I know this isn't like me; I know it's not normal. Other people are going out and doing things: why am I too terrified to do this?

The pain and distress that this fear evoked in me was shattering – both physically and psychologically exhausting. The intensity of the emotion, the speed at which it would roar into life and take over all of me, and the extended time it would take before it even began to subside a little bit, was overwhelming. I had never experienced anything like this. I couldn't manage it and I couldn't make it stop. Rapidly, it took over my life, day after day.

The only way I felt like I could cope was to not 'provoke' the fear. If I was careful, my fire-breathing dragon would lie smouldering in my guts, and I would do anything to avoid disturbing this partial slumber, frightened of the consequent roaring of terror that would come back into my life. So I became more scared of my intense, uncontrollable emotions and tip-toed through my life. Fearful of so many things, I avoided more and more situations. In combination with being unable to wear a mask, I increasingly withdrew from social interactions. Too scared and worried to meet anyone indoors, I retreated behind my front door and continued to only meet up with a few trusted people for a walk outside. My partner was the only person I was able to allow into my house, or get physically close to, and he became an essential life raft in my increasingly turbulent emotional sea.

I went from being a consummate 'hugger' of friends and family, to now not being able to bear to be near people. The pandemic significantly exacerbated the instinctual vulnerability I felt straight after my accident. Even back in those early days, I can remember trying to go out, shrinking away from people, noise, cars or trains, scared that I might accidentally get hurt in some way. Now, with the threat of Covid-19 as well, the closer anyone came towards me, the more I would instinctively withdraw, edging to one side, trying to protect myself from perceived harm. Worst of all was anywhere where I felt like I could not escape, especially any enclosed spaces like rooms, corridors, or even narrow pavements. I would feel the panic rising exponentially, a fear-induced 'flight' instinct prompting my adrenalin to rush through me, and I would often physically try to flee, running blindly away with no idea of where I was heading, just keeping going until I was far away from people and would slowly feel safe again.

[Rudi]
I've never been much of a hugger, and my social default is preferring to be on my own, rather than with a crowd. However, in the wards, I am in close proximity to people all the time. We sit together in the gym, waiting or doing the morning handover. The rest of the day, I go from bay to bay, from bed to bed. The people I see represent the full kaleidoscope of humanity. Different backgrounds, different personalities, different histories. But all are here because they have sustained a brain injury. Some also have Covid-19. Many are very lonely, craving someone to talk to, someone to be near, even if they say nothing. Family or friends could not visit because of the obvious risks. Many patients had not seen their loved ones for weeks or even months. Some wanted me to sit on their beds and invited me to do so. Many reached out and touched my arms. Some asked before they did. Many asked if they would see me again. The loneliness was palpable. The desire for human contact hung silently in the stale ward air.

One of the key drivers for my fear was to protect myself and others from harm. The frequently cited panacea of 'don't worry, what's the worst that could happen?', no longer applied in my mind. The 'worst' had happened, and not just once. I had been in a near-fatal accident, I had a debilitating, life-changing brain injury, my much-loved disabled brother had died suddenly, and a global pandemic had changed everyone's lives, causing many deaths and severe illness. I no longer had any confidence that 'everything would be alright', I felt like I had totally lost control, and had an overwhelming urge to do everything I could to stay safe and not suffer any further harm. The human instinct for self-preservation is incredibly strong, and although it can be critical in emergency situations, unfortunately, in my case, this powerful emotion was being inappropriately deployed. I became 'over-protective', both psychologically and behaviourally, and in withdrawing from life so much I began to cause myself longer-term harm in a different way. I did not realise at this point what the impact of this would be on my future mental health and ability to engage in neurological rehabilitation and adjust to my brain injury.

I was obviously not the only person to feel an increased level of stress and anxiety at this time. A number of studies have shown that there was an increase in anxiety amongst the population as a whole during Covid-19. In particular, anxiety levels were at their highest during the first lockdown, and reduced as lockdown eased in the summer of 2020, although they did not return to the national pre-pandemic level. The UK Government compiled data from national surveys and academic research to provide a comprehensive picture of the levels of anxiety in the whole population during the first two years of the pandemic. It found a variable profile of increasing and decreasing anxiety levels:

> Two sources of weekly data on levels of anxiety symptoms in the general population … Both suggest an initial trend of reducing anxiety from a high point measured early in the first national lockdown. Trends then level off through late spring and summer 2020 but remain above the best available pre-pandemic baseline. There is evidence of a further increase in average levels of anxiety between August and mid-winter 2020, but not back to the levels reported early in the first lockdown.
>
> (UK Government, 2022)

Higher levels of anxiety were also experienced by many people with a brain injury during the pandemic. In the early period of the pandemic, a significant 64% of people with a brain injury in the UK reported an increase in their anxiety (Headway, 2020). This increase in anxiety was even more significant for many people working in the health sector and other key occupations that involved close engagement with people with the virus.

(iv) Emotional Fireball

Whilst an increase in anxiety and stress was initially felt by so many people during the pandemic, these feelings gradually reduced for many as lockdown eased. This has been termed 'hedonic adaptation' – the psychological ability to bounce back after a shock event.

The effect seen on average anxiety ratings throughout the coronavirus (COVID-19) pandemic shows a similar pattern to the theory of 'hedonic adaptation' (Diener and others, 2006). When a shock event occurs, such as the impact of the coronavirus, well-being is temporarily impacted but people then quickly adapt so that well-being partially bounces back; though not necessarily to the same level as it was before the shock.

(Office for National Statistics, 2020)

This reduction in anxiety levels did not happen to me. Instead, my stress increased and my fear became overwhelming. I have subsequently asked myself why my emotions were so intense and why my stress levels stayed so high for so long. I began to learn that it was in part my cognitive difficulties in managing or moderating my emotions since my brain injury that was making the pandemic so difficult for someone like me.

It was the sheer intensity of my fear during the pandemic that was the hardest thing, along with how easily it was triggered, and how difficult it was to lower these feelings back down again. This differed significantly from my 'pre-brain injury' experience. I had previously been someone who had a reasonably healthy emotional response to most situations. Like most of us, I would on occasion get a bit stressed by work or climbing a mountain that would stretch me well out of my comfort zone, but that was usually just a short-lived emotion, well-managed and quickly resolved. Whilst not being a 'risk-taker', I was also known as a person who would take on challenging situations which would have been too much for many other people, like racing down an alpine pass on a bicycle. I used to be strong, confident, emotionally stable and able to respond appropriately to the many issues that arise in day-to-day life. I was quite capable of facing up to my fears, taking action and moving on. My emotions were usually manageable and transient. Most of all, they were proportionate to the situation I was experiencing at the time.

So what had changed? What had happened in my brain that made it so difficult for me to manage and moderate my emotions? It has been increasingly recognised that a brain injury can cause emotional issues. Some of these arise from the challenge of adjusting to the changes that happen as a result of a brain injury, such as not being able to work, whilst other negative emotions can be caused by executive dysfunction whereby changes to memory, attention or decision-making can result in cognitive overwhelm, which in turn can cause anxiety or anger. Although I had experienced all of these things, it was not this that was causing my extreme emotional response to the fear of the pandemic. For me, it was a change in my cognitive ability to limit and manage the intensity of my emotions that was the key issue, a process in the brain that I came to learn was referred to as 'emotional regulation'.

Emotional regulation relates to the capacity to flexibly modulate and control subjective experience and expression of emotions, and the reduction of emotional arousal. In ABI, there may be impairments in self-monitoring and control ... Further, emotional regulation is an important aspect of executive functioning (EF), broadly described as inter-related top-down processes promoting the control and regulation of cognition, behavior, and emotion.

(Stubberud, 2020)

Cognitive impairment in self-monitoring and control can lead to 'emotional dysregulation', and there is a growing awareness of this as a significant sequelae in people with an acquired brain injury (ABI). It is conceptualised as 'a group of difficulties in the ability to modify the intensity or trajectory of an unfolding emotion to achieve a more desirable emotional state' (Pepping et al., 2024). In my case, I have a degree of emotional dysregulation that is significant enough to challenge my ability to manage my emotions. With the increase in stress that was caused by the pandemic, my limited ability to manage the intensity of my anxiety resulted in an extremely high level of fear. This, in turn, prompted a cascade of avoidance behaviours, as I effectively locked myself away in the perceived safety of my home, reducing my social contact, resulting in a vicious negative spiral of declining mental health.

So having a traumatic brain injury meant it was much harder for me to manage the stress and anxiety associated with Covid-19. Like many complex, inter-related systems, the anxiety caused by the threat of the virus was exacerbated by my psychological stress response from my preceding traumatic experience, and the intensity of these emotions was heightened by my cognitive impairments relating to emotional regulation. My emotions were as out of control as a speeding car: my fear would escalate rapidly, the accelerator pushed to the floor, my emotional engine screaming, with no let-up, no off-switch and no gradual deceleration. At the time,

I wasn't aware of this hidden impact of my brain injury; during the pandemic, I was trying my best to just cope. Whilst I continued as best I could with my quiet time in nature, occasional meeting with friends outdoors for a 'walk and talk', photography and support from my partner, the importance of regular rehabilitation in helping me cope during these difficult times came to the fore.

(v) Help: The Role of Rehab

As the pandemic progressed, I felt like I was only just hanging in there. Confused by the effects of my brain injury and my cognitive difficulties, exhausted by days of neurological fatigue and overwhelmed by intense emotions, I needed professional help. My weekly neuropsychological rehab sessions with Rudi became a veritable port in the storm, and I was extremely grateful for his support.

As the pandemic continued, we shifted from telephone calls to online discussions using the now ubiquitous Teams meetings. This was a significant improvement on the more anonymous phone calls, as we could see each other, albeit only on screen and our upper bodies. Subtle messages were still lost, even with these more personal interactions, for example, the signs of stress and anxiety in a twitching leg. As my rehabilitation progressed, I also sent in regular written updates, which I emailed to Rudi in advance of our sessions. In addition to these written thoughts, I also included drawings covering in more detail many of the things that I struggled to find the words to explain, and often used colour to communicate emotions as well as information. Advanced preparation facilitated this much more deliberative and reflective practice and enabled me to develop deeper insights into the challenging effects of my brain injury.

Despite some technical difficulties and the above-mentioned limitations of these telehealth approaches, there were also some significant practical benefits of having online sessions. As the pandemic continued, these were critical in providing me with much needed continuity of neuropsychological rehabilitation and, most importantly, offered a safe and secure opportunity to engage without the risk of catching Covid-19 or of passing it on to others. It also provided some practical benefits by removing the need to travel to the clinic, therefore reducing the cognitive demands of driving and navigating. The positive practical aspects of the introduction of telehealth approaches during the pandemic have also been noted in qualitative research interviews with people with an acquired brain injury:

> Participants appreciated the efficiency and conveni-ence compared to in-person appointments, which saved time for patients and healthcare providers. Video calls were generally accepted as more satis-factory, as they allow healthcare practitioners and patients to view facial expressions and provide a sense of human connection. Eliminating the need for transportation to appointments was another advan-tage, especially for those living in rural areas. A par-ticipant noted how online appointments required less energy to prepare for.
>
> (Wong et al., 2022)

After six months of telephone and online sessions, in early September 2020, Rudi suggested a 'home visit' to check in on how I was doing, providing an in-person opportunity that could offer more insight and inter-action than a phone call. Although welcome, this offer prompted a significant increase in my stress about the virus and the potential risks to both myself and Rudi. Since the start of the pandemic, no-one had been allowed in my house, apart from visits from my partner under very strict conditions, which even then caused me extreme anxiety. Ever since my accident, I had felt vulnerable and reluctant to have any visitors, triggered by some kind of subconscious response, and this sensa-tion had become even more apparent since the start of Covid-19. I had changed significantly, as a result of the combination of the trauma from my accident and the effects of my brain injury, from an outgoing social indi-vidual with a permanent 'open door' where I welcomed friends to stay at any time, to a reclusive hermit. My home had become both a fortress and a prison, keeping everyone out and locking myself inside.

Panic set in about Rudi's visit. How was I going to manage this? How can I keep him safe? How can I keep myself safe? I do not have a large house nor an exten-sive garden, and I have neighbours close by on either side. The practicalities of safe social distancing, venti-lation and privacy made planning for this clinical visit a real challenge. Tape measure in hand, I mapped out seating positions in my living room at least three metres apart. Regardless of the weather, I planned to open the patio doors at both ends of the room to maximise venti-lation and leave the front door open to create a draught down the stairs. I was concerned about what the neigh-bours might hear with the doors open, as my usual neu-rorehabilitation discussions were strictly confidential.

In addition, I was particularly sensitive about this being my home – my private space, filled with personal items and photos. It was not a clinic, and having someone in my home who had been trained in psychological observation left me feeling as exposed as a tortoise popping its head out from beneath its protective shell. What would my home say about me? Did it look like I was managing to cope, was it suitably tidy and organised?

The hardest part was my guilt about not being able to cope with wearing a face mask. As I've described before, my initial attempts at wearing a mask had prompted the most distressing flashbacks. Even thinking about putting one on would leave me shaking and sweating, trying to contain my increasing anxiety. Despite knowing that I had not been in close social contact with anyone else, I still felt overwhelming guilt at not being able to wear a mask for Rudi's home visit, potentially putting him and his other patients at risk through what I perceived as my weak and selfish behaviour. Over time, it would be a hard lesson for me to learn that all of us, no matter how psychologically robust and competent we might feel, can, under specific circumstances, be overruled by deep-rooted, powerful and overwhelming emotions and visceral memories that exist at a level beyond that of our conscious minds.

Unsurprisingly, given all the above issues and challenges, this home visit was not a comfortable or relaxed session. The discussion was stilted and my anxiety became quite significant. I have little recall of what we talked about, although I remember trying to keep my shaking legs still whilst I tried to subdue an urge to flee. It was in many ways a 'success' in that we both worked hard to ensure that we minimised any risk of viral transmission, and for the first time, I overcame my fear enough to allow someone to enter the 'safe space' in my home. As such, it was a testament to the trust I felt in Rudi, a trust that I had not extended to anyone other than my partner, not even to my family or close friends, and in that way, it was a prime example of a strengthened therapeutic bond. However, there remains a question for me about the benefit of such a visit, despite my support and agreement for it to go ahead. Did it prompt me to face up to and challenge some of my increasing avoidance behaviours? Or did it back-fire and lead to an even more significant retreat behind closed doors?

[Rudi]
My experience of the preparation for Sue's home visit mirrors what Sue described above. Every home visit was a very difficult individual decision to make, every time, and especially so regarding Sue, knowing her anxiety around Covid-19. Each time the decision to do (or not) a home visit was an attempt to balance immediate risk (passing on the virus) with longer-term benefits (mental health). The risk to others related to them coming in contact with a clinician whose work environment of in-patient wards, including isolation wards, out-patient clinics, and then home visits, resulted in cumulative potential exposure to Covid-19. The other factor to consider was that the mental health benefits to in-person (or clinic-based) psychological interventions are never immediate, and often things 'get worse before they get better'. However, we also know that mental health difficulties tend to worsen when people become socially isolated.

Social isolation and loneliness are fertile grounds for anxiety, depression and withdrawal to enter a very serious downward spiral in a person's mental health. Per implication, for many people the pandemic resulted in social isolation, economic hardship and loss of purpose. These were the factors that needed balancing and counterbalancing to make the best personalised decision for every person in our care during the pandemic. In Sue's situation, whilst we maintained some momentum with her rehab by using Teams and the written material, as well as drawing, I was feeling deeply concerned that long-term isolation could make matters much worse for Sue, thinking about the future, say two or more years down the line. It was time to try and balance the discomfort of 'now', with the potential damage of 'later'. I remember doing absolutely everything I could to make sure I was 'good to go', and able to ensure her safety as best as possible before driving off, and parking outside Sue's house. Maybe in a future without Covid-19 we cannot yet imagine, today would be the first step to help make sure that future can be embraced as best as possible by Sue.

Looking back now from that future, whilst my 'Covid-19 tour' was certainly very ordinary and low-level – compared to, say, those clinical colleagues who worked long, unrelenting shifts in A&E or ITU, day in, day out, – there was still intermittent, but significant potential exposure for me to manage. I did not work from home or make much use at all of digital working during the pandemic. Being a clinician doesn't make one 'special'. The risk to me was the same, of course, as for almost all the people I cared for in the community, who often showed enormous courage. Parcels had to be delivered, boilers fixed, and shopping checkouts staffed. As a clinician, I of course knew, and fully understood my personal risk

factors, including, for example being older, and not hav-
ing antibodies (based on an early pandemic blood test
for antibodies). Once we knew more about the virus and
its transmission, as well as the arrival of regular test-
ing, risk could be assessed more objectively and very
frequently, as well as a little bit more effectively, but by
no means absolutely. There was always a niggling sense
of doubt; every cough like a potential brown envelope
containing bad news landing in your letterbox.

We are all human and fear severe illness. It is often
said that clinicians tend to suppress any thoughts around
this, for example, by believing 'illness is something that
happens to other people'. That's not quite true. Whilst
I have been very lucky to have always been calm by
nature, as clinicians, we do worry. Interestingly though,
when anxiety did arise during the pandemic, not all of
it was about our health. As a clinician, it is our ultimate
fear to do harm to our patients – primum non-nocere.
We were very anxious that we would pass on Covid-
19 to those in our care. That did sometimes keep me
awake at night. On the other hand, isn't doing nothing
also harmful? The desire to help others, whether that
is someone who asks for directions, delivering a food
parcel to someone who cannot go out, or a patient in
a hospital ward, is part of what makes us human, irre-
spective of who we are as individuals.

Unfortunately, my avoidance behaviours continued to
escalate, not as a result of this home visit, but rather due
to the escalation of my increasingly desperate drive to
find a way to control my exposure to Covid-19 and protect myself from harm. However, this presented a potential challenge in the event that I might need medical

treatment at any point (regardless of cause). Not being able to go inside any building where there might be other people would make future hospital appointments very difficult. In light of this, and as a critical element of my rehabilitation, Rudi suggested that I tried a supported visit to the clinic at the North Wales Brain Injury Service.

[Rudi]
I remember the decision to invite Sue to the unit as part of the therapeutic work to reduce the avoidance of being anywhere there might be Covid-19 (which is basically everywhere except home). This had now become an important obstacle not only to rehab, but also essential activities like, for example, attending hospital appointments for the remaining difficulties related to the injuries Sue sustained in the accident. Getting the unit ready for a visit was a priority, including 'clearing the traffic' prior to Sue's arrival. It was a nice day, and I was able to keep the windows of the room we were going to use wide open for airing. Unfortunately, I had to wear PPE, but that was unavoidable. Besides the repeated exposures, which is just part of the approach to reduce anxiety and avoidance, my main memory of the appointment is the huge respect I felt for Sue being so courageous, her bravery and tenacity like that of an ultrarunner who has already 'hit the wall' several times, but continues, nevertheless. It was bravery I had not seen before during the pandemic. Because it was relatively simple for people to avoid going to high-risk Covid-19 environments and experience instant, reinforcing relief from any anxiety; what Sue managed to do that day was truly remarkable.

I was extremely grateful for the effort that he made to ensure that this visit was achievable, arranging a quiet time at the clinic so that I would encounter no other people, and ensuring that full protective measures and ventilation were in place. Initially, when I met Rudi at the clinic, I found seeing someone in PPE disturbing as it reduced my ability to see a lot of facial expressions; in particular, the positivity of a simple smile. It also connected to my subconscious memories of the PPE worn by critical care consultants in the major trauma unit at the hospital after my accident. The enclosed corridor and room prompted a panic attack in my first attempt, a distressing experience that I was reluctant to repeat. However, the essence of rehabilitation is to provide supported interventions to help a person overcome their challenges, so with Rudi's encouragement, I tried again and again, and with repetition, this activity became achievable and the visit to the clinic was a success.

This combination of anxiety about Covid-19, the limits to non-verbal communication associated with PPE, and its interaction with the cognitive impacts of a person's brain injury, have been noted as a challenge for clinical practice in hospitals during the pandemic:

> When seeing patients, anxiety about Covid-19 can influence their presentation over and above that normally associated with their brain injury. In the ward environment, and for some community-based consultations, this anxiety can be exacerbated by the challenges associated with wearing PPE, which prevent the clinician from building a calming, therapeutic rapport. At the most basic, but crucial level – they cannot see our smile.
>
> (Coetzer, 2020)

Overall, for me, the changes to the delivery of neurorehabilitation sessions because of the pandemic represented
a complex mix of preferences and challenges. The swift
introduction of telephone and online sessions allowed
continuity of care, offered greater safety, reduced risk
and removed the demands of travel. However, these
approaches also reduced the level of therapeutic connection and limited the interactive sharing of more
multi-dimensional communication. In contrast, the
benefits of in-person engagement, including building a
more in-depth therapeutic bond and being able to see
another person's expression along with other forms
of non-verbal communication, were lost and attempts
at home-based or in-person hospital visits were over-
shadowed by extremely high levels of anxiety about the
virus and deep-rooted feelings of threat.

[Rudi]
*During the pandemic, I had never before in my career
seen such a chaotic mix of fear, depression, panic, confusion, resignation, absurdity, bravery, exhaustion,
camaraderie, kindness, sadness, relief, shock, calmness,
sorrow, denial and much more. At the time of writing
this book with Sue, I caught myself distractedly looking at an electronic photo frame on a bookshelf when,
like an uninvited guest, one of my 'pandemic photos'
flashed up on the display. Instantly, a sense of disbelief
and a realisation 'it really happened' flashed into my
brain in perfect sync with the photo frame, before the
image disappeared back into history, where it belongs.
Sometimes, the images come back even when I am far,
far away from the photo frame. Drawing upon our jour-
nals and photographs, our memories and experiences*

from both sides of the 'virtual clinic desk' are shared throughout this book, which explores and reflects on the broader mental health impact of the pandemic. Next, we will discuss loss, grief, identity and despair during the pandemic, among other mental health impacts.

(vi) Loss and Grief

In early September 2020, my partner and I decided to grab the opportunity of the easing of lockdown restrictions and visit our respective parents. Both of us had older parents in their 80s living far away in other parts of the UK, and although they were all robust, strong, independent individuals, we had been worried about them and the increased risk that elderly people faced from the virus.

For me, this was compounded by my concern for my mum due to the loss of my youngest brother. My mum had been my brother's carer every day of his life, for 47 years. Whilst his sudden death had devastated all of us, this was especially the case for my mum, who had lived with him and cared for him in every way. It is a testament to her strength and determination that she coped so well when the pandemic lockdown began, only six months after losing my brother – especially as she now had to adjust to living alone. Along with my sister and my other brother, we did what we could to support my mum within the restrictions and limitations of the lockdown. I called my mum every day, sharing our experiences of daily life and sometimes doing a video call with her whilst I was walking on the beach or up in the mountains, seeing the wild ponies that live on the hills. It became our 'virtual' way of going out together for the day. My mum embraced the online communication benefits of smartphones and we exchanged frequent messages and photos. These daily calls benefited both of us, helping to alleviate some of the isolation of lockdown, and I was immensely proud of my mum's strength and courage in coping with her grief and loss despite the most unbelievably difficult circumstances of the pandemic.

These forthcoming family visits were so important as it was the first opportunity that my partner and I had had to see our parents since the start of the pandemic. Covid-19 was still with us so we had to take certain precautions, arranging to stay in my sister's motorhome when visiting my mum, and renting a cottage near my partner's parents. Despite my continuing anxiety about being with other people indoors, we had a wonderful time. Blessed with good weather, we sat in the garden, played with numerous family dogs, and went for short walks in the countryside. Sharing memories, seeing my mum, and finally overcoming my overwhelming fear of being physically close to other people and giving her a hug goodbye: these simple but poignant experiences meant so much and have a very special place in my heart.

Tragically, the following week my mum suddenly passed away from an unexpected health condition. After a desperate drive with my partner across the UK, I was able to get to the hospital to be with her, along with my sister and brother. To add to the grief, it was also exactly a year since my little brother had suddenly passed away in the same hospital. This book is not the place to discuss our private family grief, but losing our mum was devastating for my sister, remaining brother and me. She was the pivotal person in all our lives, and we were utterly lost without her. Both my mum and my little brother showed incredible courage throughout their lives, dealing with the overwhelming challenges of living with severe disability and caring for a loved one with a life-long condition, but they both still approached life with positivity and laughter. They will always be my greatest inspiration and motivation to overcome the odds, with compassion and love, and to live life in the best possible way.

Anyone who lost a loved one during the pandemic knows of the extra emotional and practical difficulties this presented. The restrictions within the hospital, mask wearing and who was allowed to be with other people outside of specific 'bubbles' – all these things made it even harder in the face of unbelievable loss and grief. Unsure of whether or not we were allowed to be together in light of the ever-changing regulations, strictly limited in terms of funeral arrangements, we coped the best we could.

[Rudi]
It is impossible for me to fully comprehend the devastating loss Sue suffered during the pandemic. It is crucial that clinicians always remain truthful, not only in the factual, knowledge sense, but also with regard to emotions. We should never say to someone, 'I know how you feel', if we don't. I felt enormous compassion for what had happened to Sue. However, I cannot claim that I knew the exact emotions Sue must have been experiencing during that awful time for her. All I could do was be available to Sue and present in the moment when we were in sessions. I was very fortunate in that I had not experienced the loss of a family member during the

pandemic. It would be fundamentally dishonest to say that I know how that loss feels, and a terrible strategy for maintaining a therapeutic relationship.

Although the summer of 2020 had offered a hiatus in the restrictions of the pandemic, by September, the number of cases of Covid-19 had begun to rise again. It soon became clear that we were facing a 'second wave' that would grow to become more severe than the terrible first wave that we had experienced earlier in the year. The UK started to introduce 'local lockdowns', focusing on applying restrictions to specific areas which had significant outbreaks of cases. This resulted in a 'Tier System' with different places being designated as either Tier 1, Tier 2, Tier 3, etc., all with their own rules. This created a geographical patchwork of differing regulations across the country. For many people, this meant that they might be living under 'unrestricted' conditions, whilst the friends and families in another area might be subject to significant limitations on social contact and travel. The situation quickly worsened, and by mid-September, the 'rule of six' was re-introduced, limiting social mixing to only a few people.

These new and constantly changing regulations made coping with the loss of my mum and the practicalities of bereavement very challenging. With my sister and remaining brother, we tried our best to manage everything at a distance. On top of my grief, my limited cognitive capacity was constantly overloaded by processing important paperwork and making appropriate arrangements. Although my neurological fatigue increased significantly, I didn't want to leave this all to my sister and brother, who were also trying to cope with their grief.

For someone like myself with a brain injury, it can be extra difficult to manage such life-changing events as family bereavement, given my cognitive impairments and pre-existing fatigue. In addition to the effect of my brain injury, coping with the death of my mum was made even harder by the different geographical restrictions of everchanging lockdowns. These made it difficult for my remaining family to get together in the normal way when faced with such a loss. I am grateful for the incredible support I had from my partner, family, close friends and good colleagues during this time. I also appreciated Rudi's compassion and the continuity of my rehab sessions, which helped to provide some degree of structure in a sea of despair.

(vii) Losing my Identity

On top of everything else that had happened over the two years prior, this now meant that life had got too much for me. I felt that I had lost everything: my mother and brother – two of the people I had loved most in the world; my cognitive capabilities as a result of my brain injury; my role as a researcher and my ability to join in with my friends and take part in the activities I used to enjoy. A vast emptiness filled me, creating a void in my sense of self and my place in the world. It is impossible to find the words to describe this psychological sense of loss of who I was, and my consequential inability to find a way forward to become a new person. I would walk alone for hours, feeling hollow and empty inside, devoid of any understanding of myself and what direction to take in life. I was completely and utterly lost. I turned inwards more and more, often writing in my journal in the hope of finding an answer through reflection and deliberation.

Sue's Journal October 6, 2020: LOST
How can I move forward when I don't know which way to go?
There is no signpost, no map, no direction home.
I am lost in myself, lost in my life, lost in the world.
Too scared to move forwards, too scared to go alone.
Too scared to find my way to a new home.
I need to take a step, a single step, into the unknown.
There are many cliffs lurking in the mist.
Wrong directions, hidden pitfalls.
But I have to try to find a way. I cannot stay.
I need a new home.

There is an extensive body of research on the effect that a brain injury has on an individual's sense of identity. Much of this research cites many aspects, including loss of occupation, changing family roles, loss of friends, and inability to take part in previously valued social and leisure activities. Like many people with a traumatic brain injury, when I had my accident, I lost more than I could have possibly imagined.

Yet in addition to these tangible attributes, I experienced an indescribable, invisible 'feeling' inside me. I have no words to properly explain this sensation, beyond that of an awful hollow emptiness when I psychologically reached inside myself, trying to get an understanding of who I now was. To feel nothingness, a lack of any solid sense of my identity to get a grasp of, is a scary, isolating, unbelievable experience. I felt that there was nothing inside me that said 'this is who I am, this is how I do things, this is how I can cope'. My sense of 'me' was absent, in every possible way. This feeling left me utterly bereft and I grieved for the person that I used to be, the person I no longer was, the person that I had lost. Looking back, it felt like during that 'non-existence time' of unconsciousness when my accident happened, that the person I had been, the very essence of who I was, had been taken and replaced by a new person, almost like a new-born, without any sense of identity, who I did not know. I looked the same on the outside, and to begin with, I thought I still was the same in many ways, but my sense of 'me' was missing, the person I knew, the person I thought I was, had gone.

[Rudi]
Thinking back now, while not immediately apparent at the time, and not in response to the loss of a family member, the person I was, little by little, changed during the pandemic. Some of these changes were good, some not so good. On the positive side, although the pandemic was the hardest chapter of my NHS career, in many ways it was also the best. Uncurtailed by unnecessary bureaucracy, we could just relentlessly do what we were trained to do. Less forms, less meetings, less of the 'now let me think, this is literally the 21st time I am doing this training that has no bearing on my clinical knowledge and skill' moments (meaning hours). The workload did have some unintended consequences though, fatigue being a big one. If almost all your work

is with humans who are experiencing trauma and despair, inevitably, that has an effect on your own psychological well-being. Fatigue was, of course, not only the result of being overworked, but also other factors such as Covid-19 illness, or emotional burnout, to name just two.

A more slowly evolving negative outcome revealed itself a bit later. I noticed that I had become a more cynical, less forgiving, and more judgemental person regarding clinicians' commitment to patient care. Or at least, as I subjectively perceived a colleague's commitment to do the in-person work 'in the trenches' we all should be doing. My anger about this was subtle and would manifest in my inner thoughts, such as 'I never saw you in the wards', or 'if you didn't provide support from a safe distance to us frontline staff and came to help us in the trenches, we would all be less exhausted'. It is not something I am proud of, and I wish I could change it. Unfortunately despite being aware of this problem, to this day I find a wave of irritation creeping up on me when, for example, I asked someone, 'Did you assess Mr. X, and how did you find them, and the ward?', only to be met by a break in eye contact, followed by a long, complicated explanation of why they did in fact not assess them. Afterwards, I felt guilty and tried to remind myself that we all have our fears.

One amazing gift the pandemic gave me was to learn to truly appreciate being alive, and look after my body again. As a younger man, I loved sport and took part in a variety of sports, which I loved, except running, which I have always passionately hated! In the pandemic, I became very aware of how incredibly tough-but-fragile we are physically. To be alive and able to move around freely whilst working in a sea of those who no longer had this gift, made me appreciate being alive very intensely, throw all caution to the wind and embrace life. Walking and hiking in Snowdonia was wonderful, but soon that was not enough of a fix. I started running (and confirmed that I still hated it 30 years later!). But then, despite my age, something 'clicked' about how precious life is, and I took up trail running (which is hard but wonderful), climbing (if you are afraid of heights, climb up stuff), bouldering, swimming, high impact training (HIT) and even (weather permitting) 'beach rugby'. I am a different person now, thanks to the pandemic.

Some of the less good changes in who I am now have also influenced my personal life. Despite being more of a loner anyway, I did try to reconnect socially after the isolation of the pandemic, but I failed to form a new close friendship. I am seen as a 'difficult', emotionally detached, selfish person now. To be fair, the pandemic is probably not the main villain in this saga of who I became. Instead, the correct formulation is, 'a more difficult person now than before'. Nevertheless, I try to forgive myself by reminding myself of the three main pandemic-related personal positive outcomes, as I subjectively see them. The pandemic was the stimulus for me to grab life by the scruff, exercise and take up activities I thought were not possible anymore. Secondly, the pandemic taught me more than any university training programme ever could about the importance of being compassionate and kind towards patients who are experiencing the type of suffering after a brain injury, which we don't really understand. If only I could also be that to others around me. The third positive outcome is that if someone were to ask me what I did during the pandemic, I can look them in the eyes and straight away give them a one-line answer. If I couldn't, it would now be too late for me to travel back in time to reverse that missed opportunity. And that would have crushed me.

That loss wasn't as simple as a change in the things I could do. Of course, I missed being able to race up the mountains, or buzz with ideas at an international conference, or join my friends for a weekend away. However, rather than just the loss of these activities themselves, it was my inability to do so many things that affected my sense of self through the stripping from my identity aspects that I had felt were such an integral part of me. I no longer felt strong, confident, energetic, independent, a leader and supporter of others, in control of my own destiny. Instead, now I felt vulnerable, weak, dependent, fatigued and unable to help myself, let alone support others.

Losing firstly my brother and then my mum, along with my fear of Covid-19, all added to my loss of identity from my brain injury. I was no longer a sister that had helped support my brother for all those years; I was no longer a daughter that had a mother as a central hub in life. Worst of all, in a very psychologically mixed up way, I felt that my new, brain-injured 'weak' self had not been strong enough to protect them, to save them. I could not stop these awful things from happening. The vulnerability that I had felt from the very start after my accident was exacerbated by this, and on top of it all was the feeling that I could not protect myself or my loved ones from Covid-19. My previous mantras of 'mind over matter' and 'you can't change what happens, but you can change your attitude' seemed unbelievably trite and simplistic. How naïve I had been to believe such things could be achieved easily. I became painfully aware of how I had assumed that a supposed mental strength was enough to overcome some of the immense challenges so many people experienced in their lives.

Losing your sense of self makes it very difficult to move forward to a better place, psychologically and practically. Whilst there is a frequent narrative in the context of brain injury around the shift from the 'old me' to a 'new me', there is little discussion of the veritable wasteland of the in-between period of a 'non-me'. Existing in this no-man's land for so long was incredibly hard. Many of my rehabilitation sessions with Rudi would focus on techniques and discussions to explore my values, and the more inherent aspects of life that would transcend specific activities and be transferable to more appropriate interests. I would try my best to move forward, to think positively, to imagine a 'new me' doing different things that would be compatible with my brain injury and my limited capabilities. I had ideas, potential options, but I could not feel these things as part of me. I could 'talk the talk' but not 'walk the walk', and even less make use of these suggestions to help build a new sense of identity. My energy, my passion for life, was totally lacking. Nothing felt like 'me' anymore, no matter how hard I tried. In fact, the harder I tried, the worse I felt. I was trying to force a 'new me' into life, rather than letting myself evolve naturally.

The challenge of exploring new opportunities was significantly impacted by the pandemic. So much of society shut down during lockdown and even after the easing of restrictions, significant aspects of life were very limited. It was difficult to consider starting a new activity or to try re-joining certain parts of my life in a managed way when there was so little opportunity. Prior to Covid-19, it is likely that my rehabilitation would have included trying to take part in certain activities in an iterative, progressive way. This was no longer an option – my office was completely closed, cinemas were shut, and gatherings of more than six people were not allowed. It was not just the regulations that limited my options. As previously described, psychologically I was now too scared to even consider going to the majority of places, and had great difficulties in being around more than one or two people at a time.

Within this restricted social and psychological context, it is unsurprising that my ability to develop a new identity was so challenging. However, my rehab sessions with Rudi were still critical in helping me manage during this awful, empty time. Focusing on what I could do, I would concentrate on ensuring that I tried to get out for a walk once a day. If my fatigue wasn't too bad, I would attempt a short run. My weekly updates for discussion with Rudi soon came to resemble an exercise diary! However, this served an important purpose in providing a degree of structure in my daily life, and recording my activity in terms of miles or times helped me feel that I was making some progress in my recovery.

Unfortunately, ultimately this was not enough. My loss of self-identity had become a complex mix of the effect of my brain injury, my grief about my brother and mum, my overwhelming fear and anxiety about the virus, my inability to work and my social withdrawal, and the total upheaval in society due to the pandemic. Nothing was the same and I did not understand who I was any more, or how to rebuild my life. I had reached the stage where just existing day to day was all I could manage. Life began to get too much for me, and as we moved into winter, the darkness descended not just outdoors, but in my heart and my mind.

(viii) Darkness and Despair

Despite my best efforts and the unwavering support of my partner, along with regular rehab sessions with Rudi, by the winter of 2020, I felt that I was living in a desolate grey landscape, devoid of hope and future opportunity. On top of my neurological fatigue, cognitive overload, grief at the loss of my mum, the virus began to rear its ugly head again.

Regulations continued to differ across the different countries of the UK, with Wales, England and Scotland introducing different restrictions. Faced with the rapid increase in cases, Wales introduced a 'firebreak' lockdown on October 23 for several weeks. Although this helped by temporarily reducing the exponential increase in cases, it could not stem the tide. In November 2020, England introduced its national lockdown, and people were restricted to only seeing the people within their own 'support bubble'.

The second wave was advanced and cases continued to rise quickly as we approached Christmas in 2020. As the pandemic continued, the intention to allow up to three households to mix over the festive period was limited to try to avoid overwhelming the NHS. In response, on December 20, a new Tier 4 was introduced in certain areas, which limited people to only mixing with their own households. Other areas were permitted to mix with up to two other households only, forming a 'Christmas Bubble' for one day. As before, there were different regulations in Wales, England and Scotland, with all of Wales being in the equivalent of Tier 4.

[Rudi] Christmas Eve, December 24, 2020
My journal inscription in grey pencil letters simply reads: 'Today was my last day at work before going on leave for two weeks. I felt guilty in a strange way when I left the ward, perhaps seeing all the patients who won't be able to go home for Christmas, made me feel sad and guilty'. Apologies for the poor grammar, the above is taken directly from the journal. A sole photograph I took on December 24, 2020 (at 16:39) is of the whiteboard on the green wall of the ward's gym (which doubles up as our communal office). It is a cartoon of an imaginary Christmas scene. The characters drawn clearly are some of us dressed in hospital garb, with exaggerated depictions of some of our personal 'trademarks' (for example, outrageous socks). In the background, there is a house, a person just visible through a small window, shouting, 'help!' At the left-hand top of the cartoon, the most dominant feature of the drawing, in big, bold, bright, red letters: 'Nadolig Llawen!!'.

Unfortunately, as the rules changed over and over again, the cognitive load of understanding and remembering the regulations in my area (and those for my family and friends in different places), began to cause me greater confusion. Where was I allowed to walk? How far? How often? Who could I see? Where was my county boundary? How far was five miles away from my house? What was meant by this 'Tier 1' or 'Tier 2'? Who could be in a bubble, were they from different houses? Making decisions about where I could go, who I could see, and whether that was the same this week compared to last week, blew any semblance of routine out of the window. As fast as I tried to settle into a new way of doing things, the rules would change again, and my brain would struggle to keep up with what all that would mean for both me and others.

For someone like myself with a brain injury, this was very challenging. 'Switching' from one set of rules to another was much harder cognitively than when everything stayed the same, no matter how limiting that might have been. When my brain gets overloaded, it just shuts down, like a computer when faced with repeated commands that come too fast for it to process. So all these changes meant that my neurological fatigue increased significantly during this period, and I spent many hours unable to move or do anything, lying silently on my own with the curtains closed in a darkened room.

My fear and anxiety rose in line with the increase in cases, and my sense of despair deepened. Isolated from family and friends, lacking the cognitive ability to distract myself by focusing my brain on work, and devoid of purpose and meaningful activities, depression fell over me like a heavy, dark shroud.

Sue's Journal November 30, 2020
I phoned the Samaritans last night. I didn't know what else to do, or where to turn. It wasn't that I was on the brink of killing myself, I just don't want to live any more. There is nothing there, nothing

left inside me. I wish I could go back in time, to the happy days. That wonderful summer of 2018 – Mum and Pete were still here, I had so much energy, I was flying up the mountains on my bike, rushing off to London for work, laughing with everyone. I want to be back there again, but I can't. I'm not me any more. I feel like the person I used to be died on the road when the car hit me; all that is left is the outer shell, my physical body with nothing left inside. Now all I feel is darkness. It is so heavy, so all-consuming, it goes on for day after day. I have no energy to try to fight it, or even to emerge. I don't even know if I want to any more. I can feel the urge to be with Mum and Pete, to leave all this dark behind me. There is no hope, no energy, no joy in life any more. I don't want to be here, I don't want go forward with this life.

I no longer thought of 'moving forwards', it took every-thing I had just to exist, using every molecule of psy-chological strength to get through the day. I could only cope with managing to get through the next minute, the next hour, to make it to the evening before another restless, sleepless night. Often, the darkness was all-encompassing for day after day, but occasionally this would lift slightly to a lighter shade of grey. It wasn't much, but it made me hang on in there.

My on-going rehab sessions were a critical life-line. Rudi had offered the option of making a referral to medical colleagues to consider medication during this time, but I did not feel that it was right for me. It wasn't that I wanted to feel such bleak, dark despair, but equally, I didn't want to mask it with drugs, fearing that all I would be doing was delaying the day when I would have to stop the medication and face my distress and grief again. In a strange way, I also didn't want to lose my grief for my mum and brother; the extent of my feeling was a tangible expression of how much they meant to me. My love for them meant that I needed to grieve, to feel their loss. My greatest fear was that taking any medication would mean that I would lose my sense that they were still with me, hearing their laughter and voices, and feeling their love. Their physical loss was bad enough, I didn't want to lose them emotionally as well.

There are a number of clear causes of my significant depression, including bereavement, Covid-19, and the impact of my brain injury on limiting my work, social life, and activities. Each of these on their own is sufficient to cause a prolonged period of negative emotions. In combination, these multiple devastating life events were overwhelming. Whilst grief is a normal human emotion, and natural after losing a loved one, this can become more complicated with repeated bereavements over a relatively short time period. It is also a complex emotion to grieve for the loss of one's self, which is what I very much experienced as a result of my brain injury. It is difficult to explain this sense of loss and grief of 'self' when to most people it appears that you are very much still here.

The effect of the pandemic was also still clearly affecting everyone. In November 2020, one in five adults in the UK reported significant depression, which was double the level from before Covid-19. Reports of depression were also much higher in certain social groups, including people with a disability (Office of National Statistics, 2020). In particular, over half of people with a brain injury (53%) reported a worsening of their depression (Headway, 2020). There was also a strong correlation during the pandemic between depression and higher levels of loneliness. For some people, the long empty days of lockdown and the subsequent lack of 'normal' socialisation during the various restrictions on activities and gathering led in some ways to an increase in 'rumination'. Rumination is a form of repetitive thinking of negative feelings and experiences, which in turn makes it difficult to move beyond these to a more positive, problem-solving attitude. I certainly found that my days were sometimes spent in this negative thought cycle. Without the distraction of other people or purposeful activities, I found it hard to break out of this.

In addition, there is also evidence that the high incidence of depression in people with a brain injury might in part be due to organic damage to the areas of the brain responsible for regulating emotions. About 50% of people with a head injury will have some form of depression in the following years, at a rate that is on average ten times higher than the general population. In a similar way to my high levels of anxiety, it is possible that the overwhelming depression that I experienced was related to the damage inside my brain. Understanding the actual mechanism behind the high incidence of depression in people like me with a TBI is still being explored. In part, it is related to the complex interaction of the various impacts of a brain injury, including impairments to cognitive functions, neurological fatigue and headaches (Kumar et al., 2018). Recent interesting research has focused on the role of post-injury inflammation in the brain in disrupting the neural pathways that control emotions. However, this work notes that the exact causes of the high levels of depression in people with a brain injury is still not clear.

> The mechanistic cause for the increased depression risk associated with a TBI remains to be defined. As TBI results in chronic neuroinflammation, and priming of glia to a secondary challenge, the inflammatory theory of depression provides a promising framework for investigating the cause of depression following a TBI.
>
> (Bodnar et al., 2018)

Although promising, with new studies currently underway on the use of pre-emptive antidepressants as soon as possible after a brain injury, there is still no comprehensive understanding of the causes of such a high level of depression in people with a traumatic brain injury. So despite the potential benefits of the use of antidepressants in not only alleviating the symptoms of depression, but also affecting the inflammatory response in the brain, it was not a treatment approach that felt right for me at that time.

So the way forward was through 'talking therapy'. It was not an easy path, nor a quick route. It was a long, hard journey, often feeling like I was going nowhere, but slowly, inch by inch, I was clawing my way back to a better place. Whilst my partner and close friends were incredibly supportive, my level of depression took me to a place of such darkness that they could no longer help me. I felt so broken, but there was nothing that my closest loved ones could do to 'fix' me. I needed professional clinical treatment and support. At this point, my regular neurore-habilitation sessions with Rudi became critical in help-ing me continue during these dark times. For a long time, literally all I could do was 'hang on', feeling that I was gripping on to life with my finger tips and just hoping to make it to the end of the day. The benefits of 'talking' were not immediately apparent, but slowly my mindset began to change. The darkness did not immediately lift, but there would be occasional breaks, little glimmers of light. These tiny seeds of positivity were carefully tended by both Rudi and myself, nurtured with compassion, and slowly they grew roots during the long, dark days of winter. Despite not seeing any immediate results, these small, tentative feelings would become apparent in the next few months. As winter drew to a close and the spring of 2021 began to emerge, there was a small glimmer of hope. There was finally a vaccine for Covid-19.

[Rudi]
We learn more from our patients than we might be aware of at the time; things textbooks cannot teach us during our clinical training. Through working with Sue, I learned about bravery to face one's deepest fears during one's darkest hours. I learned that if things could be 'fixed' immediately through talking, our jobs would require very little investment in training and that Instagram was 'a better doctor than us'. No, on the contrary, psycho-therapy is hard work and takes a lot of courage from someone to engage in that process. The small changes are not immediately apparent, meaning there is no real reinforcer. The person has to stay with what is incred-ibly painful, frightening or enraging all the time, which

requires resilience and bravery. Sue had that in abundance, and I always admired her quiet strength.

References

Armstrong, A., Brockett, B., Eustice, T., Lorentzon, A., O'Brien, L., & Williams, S. (2021). *Why society needs nature: Lessons from research during COVID-19.* Environment Agency; Forest Research; Natural England; Natural Resources Wales; NatureScot. Crown Copywrite.

Bodnar, C. N., Morganti, J. M., & Bachstetter, A. D. (2018 October). Depression following a traumatic brain injury: Uncovering cytokine dysregulation as a pathogenic mechanism. *Neural Regeneration Research, 13*(10), 1693–1704. PMID: 30136679; PMCID: PMC6128046. https://doi.org/10.4103/1673-5374.238604

Coetzer, R. (2020). First impressions of performing bedside cognitive assessment of COVID-19 inpatients. *Journal of the American Geriatrics Society, 68*(7), 1389–1390. https://doi.org/10.1111/jgs.16561

Headway. (2020). *The impact of lockdown on brain injury survivors and their families.* Headway: The Brain Injury Association.

Kumar, R. G., Gao, S., Juengst, S. B., Wagner, A. K., & Fabio, A. (2018). The effects of post-traumatic depression on cognition, pain, fatigue and headache after moderate-to-severe traumatic brain injury: A thematic review. *Brain Injury, 32*(4), 383–394. https://doi.org/10.1080/02699 052.2018.1427888

Lassaletta, A. (2020). *The invisible brain injury.* Routledge.

Office for National Statistics. (2020). *Coronavirus and anxiety, Great Britain: 3 April 2020 to 10 May 2020.* www.ons.gov.uk/peoplepopulationandcommunity/wellbeing/articles/coronavirusandanxietygreatbritain/3april2020to10may2020.

Pepping, N., Weinborn, M., Pestell, C. F., Preece, D. A., Malkani, M., Moore, S., Gross, J. J., & Becerra, R. (2024). Improving emotion regulation ability after brain injury: A systematic review of targeted interventions. *Neuropsychological Rehabilitation*, 1–41. Advance online publication. https://doi.org/10.1080/09602011.2024.2398029

Royal College of Speech and Language Therapists. (2022). *Understanding the need for and provision of speech and language therapy services for individuals with post-COVID syndrome in the UK.* Royal College of Speech and Language Therapists.

Stubberud, J., Løvstad, M., Solbakk, A. K., Schanke, A. K., & Tornås, S. (2020). Emotional regulation following acquired brain injury: Associations with executive functioning in daily life and symptoms of anxiety and depression. *Frontiers in Neurology, 11*, 1011. https://doi.org/10.3389/fneur.2020.01011

UK Government. (2022 April). *COVID-19 mental health and wellbeing surveillance: report.* www.gov.uk/government/publications/covid-19-mental-health-and-wellbeing-surveillance-report/3-triangulation-comparison-across-surveys#introduction

Verhoeks, C., Bus, B., Tendolkar, I., & Rijnen, S. (2024). Cognitive communication disorders after brain injury: A systematic COSMIN review of measurement instruments. *Annals of Physical and Rehabilitation Medicine, 67*(6), 101870. https://doi.org/10.1016/j.rehab.2024.101870

Wong, M. M. Y., Seliman, M., Loh, E., Mehta, S., & Wolfe, D. L. (2022). Experiences of individuals living with spinal-cord injuries (SCI) and acquired brain injuries (ABI) during the COVID-19 Pandemic. *Disabilities, 2*(4), 750–763. https://doi.org/10.3390/disabilities2040052

Chapter 5

No More Change? Is This the End?

Sue Williams and Rudi Coetzer

(i) Vaccines and Virus: Hope and Despair

The development of new vaccines to protect against severe illness from the coronavirus was fantastic news. Finally, it felt that we might have a way out of this awful global pandemic. In the UK, the first vaccines were given in December 2020, initially to those most in need, including the elderly and health workers. The vaccine rollout programme continued into early 2021, with everyone being asked to get vaccinated to protect themselves and others. I waited patiently for my appointment, appreciating that there were others at much greater risk from the virus. I was fortunate that I could keep myself safe at home, waiting for my turn.

However, my fear and anxiety about being close to other people, especially in enclosed places, along with my flashbacks triggered by wearing a mask, meant that the thought of going to the vaccination centre also filled me with dread. For the first time, I needed to address my fear and find a way of managing it enough to be able to get vaccinated against Covid-19. For weeks, I tried to cope with the emotional conflict that it caused in me, an inner battle between fear and hope. My rehab sessions

DOI: 10.4324/9781003509134-8

with Rudi helped me talk through these fears, and think of strategies to overcome them. A combined tactic was put in place. Rudi wrote to my GP explaining about my brain injury and psychological difficulties, my GP contacted the health authority, who were co-ordinating the vaccine programme, and between them, a few measures were put in place to help me attend. This support made a lot of difference, I was able to wait outside away from other people (rather than join an enclosed queue). When it was my turn, I was called in directly to the vaccine desk closest to an open door. It was a spacious open hall, no hidden corners, closed doors or narrow corridors where something unexpected might suddenly appear, and only one person in the vicinity. One quick jab and short discussion, and I was in and back out again. My legs shook so much with a combination of fear, adrenalin, and relief.

However, despite the optimism of the vaccine, and the various geographical local lockdowns and restrictions, the pandemic continued to sweep across the country. January 2021 saw the peak of this second wave, with the maximum number of daily cases far exceeding that of the first wave. Consequently, a further national lockdown was put in place at the start of 2021, from January to March, with similar restrictions to the first national lockdown, although small 'support bubbles' were now permitted. This was in recognition of the mental health impacts of the continuation of social distancing and isolation. It was a strain for everyone and it felt like the virus was never going to end.

[Rudi] January 21, 2021
Working in the ward, I had seen a new admission, someone who had suffered a Stroke, rendering them

unable to speak. Despite their inability to speak, I felt we made a connection. I caught myself thinking of them a lot afterwards, including becoming acutely aware that they were quite a bit younger than myself, and that fate does not choose a time to visit us (from journal, January 21, 2021, and subsequent journal notes over the next three months). I saw them regularly over the next three months and became very fond of them. In fact, they were adored by the staff. I remember the day some of the nursing staff administering a hair-cut, a really beautiful memory to this day. I also remember their broad smiles every time I saw them. About three months since, see-ing them for the first time, I arrived at the ward, being met by ashen colleagues looking at me in disbelief. Our patient's health had suddenly taken a significant turn for the worse, and they had been moved to a side room on the ward. They were 'not expected to make it'. I was asked by my colleagues, 'Could you please go and see him? His loved one is in the room with him'.

In the dim light of the side room on the ward, they were in a pristine white bed, with some monitors occa-sionally making a beep. I introduced myself to their loved one. They were beside themselves with fear and every time the monitor made a beep, asked me, 'Is that a good sign?'. They were deeply unconscious, and I had to tell their loved one the truth. I did that in the kindest way I could under those dreadful circumstances. When I next came to the ward, I heard that they had passed away over the weekend. During the day, I walked past their bed in the cubicle where they had been for three months. There was a new patient in their bed. Later, I looked into the side room where I had seen them for the last time. It was empty. I felt an intense sadness, and somewhat broken. The next day, I was back on the ward, feeling drained and empty. I saw seven patients on the ward and then taught fourth-year medical students after work.

Unsurprisingly, as the cases of Covid-19 continued to rise, my fear and anxiety also increased. Daily reports on the news filled my mind and it seemed that the virus had the upper hand no matter what we did as a society. The second lockdown in early 2021 hit me even harder than the first. I was exhausted from the previous year, after relentless months of being scared, depressed, isolated and worried. So much had happened; I had been psychologically knocked down so many times that I no longer had the strength to try to get back up again. My brain injury meant that I struggled to manage the intensity of my emotions and I wasn't able to recover from these repeated episodes of stress, anxiety and depression. Strung out with grief for my mum and brother, but unable to see my family, this made the process of managing loss and bereavement so much harder. The restrictions also meant that it wasn't possible to see even my closest friends. My partner was the only person I would see and even that was limited; his work meant that he had to be in contact with other people, so the increased risk of catching the virus meant that there were many days when we would stay apart in our own houses. Within the restrictions of lockdown, I continued to try to go for a walk every day, despite my overwhelming fatigue. I also picked up my camera again and returned to my daily photography project as a way of keeping me going when I was on yet another lonely walk in the rain.

Despite the relief and joy of the vaccine rollout, the rise of cases in early 2021 meant it felt more like Covid-19 … lockdown … isolation … exhaustion … would it never end?

(ii) Back to Work: Intermittently

The saving grace during this time was my return to work. It had always been my 'go-to' coping mechanism during difficult times, but my brain injury meant that I had struggled to manage my work with my cognitive difficulties. My job had always been important to me. I was passionate about my research on people and the environment, and cared a lot about being able to make a contribution to achieving a positive difference in the world. I had worked for the same organisation for 15 years and was fortunate to have fantastic colleagues, many of whom were also good friends. I had always loved the intellectual energy of sharing ideas with research colleagues across the UK and internationally, often coming home exhausted, but buzzing, from a long meeting at what I used to refer to as my 'brain gym'. I was renowned at work for disappearing into a research wormhole, often emerging with a spark of energy saying 'this is *really* interesting …', a phrase that I repeated with such enthusiasm that it would provoke much laughter from my teammates. Admittedly, I was at times something of a workaholic, working long days with early starts and late nights, and burning the candle at both ends. Inevitably, occasionally I'd get a bit stressed, but this was short lived and often just gave me an extra spurt of energy. I loved my job before my brain injury, and I felt competent, professional, respected and valued.

Having to step down from work due to my brain injury was one of the hardest things to accept. Even in the first year after my accident, I tried so hard to return to work as soon as possible. Unfortunately, as soon as I returned to work, I was hit by cognitive overload, attention difficulties, confusion, stress and cumulative neurological fatigue. Despite trying my hardest, I hadn't been able to cope with work and had been on long-term sick leave throughout much of 2020. It had shattered me to not be able to do my job. It was not just a 'job' to me, although, like most people, I needed to work for a salary as I lived alone and was responsible for my household and living costs. My career meant a huge amount; it was an integral part of who I was. My sense of identity was inextricably tied to my role as a researcher, and I had spent a lifetime learning and working on the things that I cared about so passionately. If I wasn't able to do my job, what was the point in getting up every day? It wasn't enough for me to just go for a walk, or take a few photos. I needed my life to have purpose, drive and value, and I wanted to make use of my remaining intellectual capacity and regain some confidence and self-respect.

I thus wanted to try to return to work but to do so in a way that might be sustainable and not tip me over the edge again. Rehab discussions with Rudi helped me to consider my capacity, how to manage some of the challenging aspects of my job and how to balance work with neurological fatigue. I was fortunate that, as an academic, Rudi also related to the buzz of research and hopefully understood why trying to return to work meant so much to me. I knew it wasn't going to be easy or straightforward, and I was concerned that I might fail again, but trying to return to work would at least give me something else to focus on rather than death, grief and despair. It would also offer an opportunity to reduce my isolation and provide a degree of structure, purpose and social interaction (albeit only online).

Due to the Covid-19 lockdown, my employer had shut down all our offices across the country, and this continued in 2021, even after the easing of the strictest restrictions. All staff had been sent home and were now working remotely, connecting online via Teams, emails and phone calls. Occasional outdoor 'walk meetings' had been arranged by some colleagues as a way of helping overcome social isolation and improve mental health and well-being. Equally, all my previous UK and international meetings and conferences had shifted to online as well. No longer was my working world about busy offices, lots of train travel and crowded conferences. For someone like me, with a brain injury that meant I struggled to cope with busy places with lots of distractions, background conversations, and the complexity of travel, this was an unexpected bonus of the pandemic. Maybe this significant change in working practices would be enough to enable me to return to work successfully?

Working from home was definitely a crucial factor in my ability to return to work, especially as I live alone and my home is silent with no distractions. This in itself reduced my cognitive load and meant that I could concentrate exclusively on my research. If it had just been me working from home, it would not have been that easy for me to go back to my job, as I would have missed out on in-person team meetings and conferences. However, working from home now applied to virtually everyone else within my organisation and internationally. All my work meetings and conferences were now online and

I could join in with these without the additional burden of travel, which had been so difficult with my brain injury before the restrictions of the Covid-19 lockdown. So in many ways, work was now more accessible to me.

However, returning to my job with a brain injury was not as simple as just working from home. I found many things surprisingly difficult, including being unable to cope with multiple emails or online presentations. With the shift to remote working, there was a significant increase in emails at my workplace and I immediately noticed the challenges this presented. As someone who has cognitive impairments in both attention and working memory, trying to review multiple emails was impossible. My brain would rapidly become confused and overloaded, unable to comprehend which messages I had already read, what was important and which email I should focus on. Usually, I would start work by opening my laptop and reviewing my emails before focusing on prioritised research projects, but now with my cognitive impairments, I found that within about 30 minutes, my brain would crash and I would end up back in bed in a dark, silent room with my head pounding.

The other difficulty I found with the shift to remote working was online conferences, although this was more beneficial than in-person meetings in many ways. My brain could not cope with looking at the slides, whilst at the same time hearing someone speaking, especially when what the voice was saying did not completely match what was on the slides. I would find that if I listened, then I would have absolutely no recall of what had been on the slides. Equally, if I read the slides, I would have a complete absence of any knowledge of what had been said. For my brain nowadays, it was either 'read' or 'hear' – I could not do both at the same time. Adding to this cognitive confusion was the online 'chat' function, with the distraction of audience comments running in parallel to the main presentation. As online conferences continued during the pandemic, there was an increase in the development of more 'interactive' functions such as real-time polls or note-based padlets. For someone like me with a brain injury, these online functions were a fast track to cognitive overload, and I would rapidly have to drop out of meetings or just not be able to engage with these participant opportunities.

My rehab with Rudi had helped me to understand a lot more about my impairments, what caused them and how to mitigate or manage some of their effects. However, applying this knowledge to my experience at work was more complex and required a partnership approach between me, Rudi and my work colleagues. I knew what my job required and I could discuss some of this with Rudi and consider tactics that might help. I realised that with my type of brain injury, I could often only focus on just one thing, and that I could no longer simultaneously process multiple sources of information. I learned to ask for presentation slides in advance so I could read them without distraction, then during the actual presentation, I could shut my eyes, not look at the slides, and just listen to what the presenter was saying. Responding to emails was much more of a challenge, and it was not easy to find a solution to this until my employer finally provided some admin support who effectively acted as my 'email processing brain'. Needless to say, trying to work with cognitive impairments was incredibly tiring and my brain was frequently overwhelmed. It took so much more effort to do the things that used to come so

quickly and easily, and I frequently felt that I was fall-
ing further behind and unable to make an acceptable and
equal contribution to work. I am incredibly grateful for
my wonderful, supportive colleagues who offered to
help and support me in so many ways, and would kindly
say that 'an hour of my time was worth more than a day
of someone else'.

In light of this support, the shift to home working during the pandemic then offered me a real opportunity to
return to work. With most workplace activities now taking place online, this also meant I was able to take part
in many more meetings and conferences than I had been
able to do before the pandemic. It was not easy, and
I continued to get repeated periods of overwhelming
neurological fatigue that required long periods off work
to recover my cognitive capacity. However, without the
social change to working practices that were put in place
due to Covid-19, I do not think I would have been able
to return to work after my brain injury. Slowly, I felt that
I might be able to emerge from the world of darkness
and take a more active part in life again.

(iii) Covid-19 Eases, but my Fears Remain

As the peak of the second wave finally receded during
the spring of 2021, the UK eased restrictions. The government issued a 'roadmap' as the vaccination rollout
continued and we slowly began an 'exit' from lockdown.
Regulations and restrictions gave way to 'guidance' and
everyone was encouraged to act responsibly especially to
protect more vulnerable people. By May 2021, Covid-19
cases were declining significantly although the virus

was still in general circulation. As the months went by and we continued into the summer, the restrictions were eased even more. The majority of the population had been vaccinated and people returned to what to many felt like a more normal life again – seeing friends, going to pubs and restaurants, meeting up in large groups, and even a degree of international travel, although restrictions remained with a constantly changing list of 'red' countries which would require quarantine.

However, for me, life did not go 'back to normal' as regulations eased. My fear and anxiety remained at a very high level and I found it impossible to believe that it was safe to go out and be around people again. The threat of the virus still lurked in every corner, and my post-traumatic stress still caused flashbacks whenever I felt threatened by the close proximity of other people or being in any enclosed places, especially indoors. Added to my concern was a growing awareness of what had now been termed 'Long Covid'. Whilst I was reasonably confident that my respiratory and cardio systems were robust and hopefully would be able to withstand the effect of the virus, I was really worried about the effect that Covid-19 could have on the brain. Equally, it was clear that most people experienced some level of viral fatigue when they caught Covid-19, and for some this was extremely debilitating and could last for a long time.

The thought of anything adding to my existing cognitive difficulties and neurological fatigue was absolutely awful. In having a life-long condition which significantly restricts what I can do every day, for the rest of my life, I felt that I needed to do everything to make sure that I didn't catch a virus that could make these impairments even worse. 'Brain fog' kept on being mentioned in accounts of the effects of Covid-19, and for me, this felt like the virus could make my cognitive difficulties even harder to cope with. I had no idea as to whether or not I was at greater risk of getting this 'brain fog' if I caught Covid-19; my brain had a pre-existing weakness as a result of the damage it had already sustained. I could not find a clear answer to this, but as people with a 'neurological condition' had been added to the 'at risk' group and prioritised for the vaccine, it felt reasonable to assume that this might be the case.

My biggest concern was the risk of having additional viral fatigue. The hardest thing I find about my brain injury is my neurological fatigue. It is there every day, the only thing that varies is how bad it is going to be. It affects everything I do, and no matter how much I might try to 'pace myself', it isn't going to go away. I have to spend my life trying to prepare for even 'normal' activities, by planning several days of pre-rest beforehand and then days of post-activity recovery, but even with forethought, the fatigue often catches me unawares. I have to cancel activities over and over again as no matter how hard I try, my fatigue is often unpredictable. It leaves me feeling left out and isolated, and often very upset. I have lost count of the number of days I have spent under the weight of this lead blanket of fatigue, where even the smallest movement feels impossible. I hate the mornings when I wake up with what I call my 'treacle brain'; when I know that attempting anything will feel like trying to wade through sticky treacle, dragging me down and being impossible to fight through. Although I try not to think about it, sometimes I remember my pre-injury days, and I dream of the energy I used to have and the bright, light feeling this used to bring. I miss that energy so much, and I still grieve privately for what I have lost and what I know I will never regain. I would give anything to have that spark of energy again, just for one day.

Consequently, as someone who now lives with debilitating neurological fatigue, I found that the thought of catching Covid-19 and having even worse fatigue filled me with horror. Life with my brain injury was bad enough and I couldn't face it getting worse. Consequently, I felt that I would prefer to carry on avoiding people, albeit with all the associated loneliness and isolation, rather than risk catching Covid-19. It felt impossible to explain to family and friends why I was so scared of this viral fatigue. I think unless you already suffer from overwhelming fatigue (which is nothing like 'feeling tired'), then you cannot begin to understand how debilitating this can be. My fear about Covid-19 then shifted from my post-traumatic flashbacks about not being able to breathe and the dread of dying, to a constant anxiety; catching the virus could make the effects of my brain injury even worse, particularly my cognitive impairments and daily fatigue. I just couldn't cope with the risk of this – having a brain injury was bad enough.

Unfortunately, this anxiety meant that I continued to isolate myself from contact with groups of people, especially indoors, where there was limited ventilation and the risk of catching the virus was much higher. At the same time, most of my friends, colleagues and family were starting to return to a more normal life. They returned to meeting up in person, and therefore many of my previous online activities didn't happen any more. Hearing about the fun that others were now having, and how much they were enjoying being able to see each other again, made me feel even more isolated. My feelings of loneliness increased, and once again I felt left out from everyday society. The world was fast returning to normal, and I couldn't join in. In part, this was due to my heightened level of fear about the neurological and fatigue impacts of Covid-19. But it was also due to my worries that my brain could not cope with being in busy indoor places. Before Covid-19, my early experiences of trying to join in normal activities, like going to a café, had been a disaster. My inability to cope with sensory demands, attention management and decision making, meant that doing these things caused immediate cognitive overload, which resulted in overwhelming pain, nausea, confusion and distress. These were such negative experiences that I no longer felt that I could manage these activities. The combination of my Covid-19 anxiety and brain injury difficulties then felt almost like lockdown life continued. Other people were going back to normal, but I was staying isolated and reluctant to even try. It was not a good place to be, and in letting these concerns limit my activities and restrict my behaviour, I was failing to learn new techniques and test approaches to manage my cognitive difficulties.

My continuing rehab sessions with Rudi were both supportive and useful in trying to understand more about the impact of my brain injury and how to manage my fatigue. This helped to counteract my worries about catching Covid-19 and the risk of exacerbating my existing difficulties. Maybe if I learned how to adapt to my brain injury, then I would be in a much better place if I eventually caught the virus? Slowly, the discussion in our sessions evolved from a regular update on my limited solo walks to considering techniques to manage the effects of my brain injury. At no point did I feel rushed to 'improve' and could gradually take my time to understand more about my cognitive impairments and how to manage the impacts that these had on my daily life.

Although still significantly constrained by the pandemic, with constantly changing regulations and my self-imposed social isolation due to my fear of catching Covid-19, my rehabilitation began to explore possibilities for the future. It had taken me three years to get to this point. I felt terribly inadequate that it was taking me so long to progress and move forward with my rehab. Rudi assured me that everyone's journey was different, and there was no set timescale for rehabilitation. I still felt that I should try harder, make more effort to improve and constantly felt guilty that I was taking limited NHS resources by needing more on-going support, especially as we were all increasingly aware of how overloaded the NHS now was due to the critical health demands of Covid-19, with an escalating backlog of treatments and exhausted staff.

[Rudi]
The end of my journey unexpectedly and slowly crept up on me. It started with undeleting an email from a recruiter. We receive many of these emails with promises of wonderful locum opportunities or similar. I always delete them. But something about this one caught my eye, and I had another look. It transpired to be a potentially interesting opportunity, and I was curious. Only problem was that I loved the NHS (I still do!) and would leave with great difficulty if I ever did. Out of curiosity,

I contacted the recruiter (who corrected my naivety by pointing out to me that they were in fact a 'head-hunter', whatever that is). The next hurdle was to find out who the employer was; I would have to commit to an interview. To cut a long story short, several interviews later and eventually being offered the role, five months had passed. And embarrassingly, I had failed to make a decision. I must have driven them mad with all my vacillation. So, one day, walking on a deserted beach (five months since the email) I reminded myself that I cannot expect others to face uncertainty, but not do that myself. That night, I formally accepted the new role with Brainkind, a UK charity, committing myself to leaving the NHS.

In the end, things turned out okay for me. I survived the pandemic: changed, but alive, unlike many others much less lucky than I have been. I have enjoyed my new role – it is still within brain injury rehab, working with lovely colleagues, and I am still active in academia as well. I'm okay, trundling along with my inner thoughts and feelings, comfortable being mostly alone with them. Empty, wild landscapes are more beautiful than ever before, and I love hiking through these places, with not a soul in sight. I cannot really complain about life. But I still miss my NHS colleagues and the patients I saw over a period of 23 years as consultant neuropsychologist in the NHS. Some patients I remember with a clarity that is difficult to describe; some because of painful memories, some because of positive memories. Sue is one of the latter, including memories of her bravery during a time too difficult to accurately capture in words. 'Covid's over. Except it's not' (Sutton, 2025).

Rudi was a critical figure in my rehab journey, and I trusted him implicitly having discussed not only my cognitive difficulties, but also my depression and anxiety during the darkest of times over the last 18 months. Therefore, it came as a shock when in June 2021, Rudi said that he would be leaving the Brain Injury Service. This felt like a significant change to me, and I was worried about how I would cope. Rudi assured me that I would not be 'discharged' from the brain injury service just because he was leaving, and that my rehab would be taken forward by another colleague. However, when you have entrusted your most private emotions to a professional neuropsychologist, it is difficult to think about having to start again with someone new. Equally, I could only begin to empathise with the challenges he must have faced during the pandemic, and how difficult that must have been.

The life-long nature of brain injury means that it can be challenging to adapt to changes in the various professional people who provide support and care; I found it difficult when both my long-standing GP retired and my work manager. Both of these people had been significant in my 'brain injury journey', and had in many ways been on a learning curve with me. We had worked together in partnership to try to understand my difficulties, especially in the first year after my accident, before I was able to access rehabilitation support with the North Wales Brain Injury Service. Their support had been very much appreciated, and I missed them more than I expected when they retired.

In particular, the nature of having a brain injury meant that I had to learn to share and discuss many of my confusing cognitive difficulties, along with my inner fears and vulnerabilities. It is private and personal, and requires a significant amount of both time and trust. There is also so much complex detail in what is experienced with a brain injury, and often it is difficult to explain these things quickly. After so many rehab sessions with Rudi, I felt that I had been able to build a strong foundation of knowledge and understanding that would act as a base to move forward to adapting to the challenges of my brain injury.

In July 2021, Rudi retired from the North Wales Brain Injury Service. Along with many others, I wanted to thank him for all his support, which had been essential in helping me to manage with a traumatic brain injury during the pandemic. I can clearly say that without his understanding, advice, empathy and support I would have been in a much harder place.

It felt daunting to think of having to meet a new neuro-psychologist, along with a new GP, and a new manager. Would these people be equally supportive? Would they understand me? How long would it take to explain everything again – weeks, months, or even years? It felt very daunting in lots of ways, and a bit of a step backwards in my rehabilitation. However, I accepted that I would have to try to start again with a new set of professional people in my life.

(iv) Tackling my Fears

Was the summer of 2021 the end of the pandemic? Had we got the better of Covid-19? Unfortunately not. The virus continued to mutate, and in December 2021, the Omicron variant spread rapidly across the world. It evaded some of the protection of the previous vaccines, and by Christmas, there was a significant increase in cases of Covid-19 throughout the UK. Initially, there was an attempt to limit the spread of Covid-19 through 'strong guidance', asking people to test, wear masks and return to social distancing. Unfortunately, this was not enough to stop the rapid rise in cases and by Boxing Day, there was a return of some of the previous restrictions, including the 'rule of six', wearing face masks and a ban on large gatherings. Slowly, cases of Omicron receded, and the UK once again returned to more nuanced guidance and the removal of restrictions in 2022.

After Rudi had moved on from the North Wales Brain Injury Service, I continued to receive support from a new neuropsychologist. However, it became increasingly clear that it was very difficult to address the challenges of my brain injury whilst I was still suffering so much with post-traumatic stress, fear and anxiety. My heightened emotional responses to my previous experiences and the pandemic meant that after two years, I still could not cope with being in close proximity to other people, especially indoors. So in 2022, I was referred to a specialist in EMDR – Eye Movement Desensitisation and Reprocessing. This type of psychotherapy has been found to reduce the symptoms of PTSD through recalling the traumatic incident in detail, whilst using side-to-side eye movements. It helps a person process the negative emotions and sensations associated with a traumatic memory that have become 'stuck' and have failed to be properly stored as a 'past' event in the brain. It is recognised as a valid technique by the National Institute for Health and Care Excellence (NICE) for the treatment of PTSD.

Despite my scepticism about how on earth this could possibly work, I wanted to give it a go. By now, I very much wanted to stop being so scared and be able to go out and be with people again. It was a long and often very difficult process, despite having a very experienced and supportive psychologist. One challenge, which made it a bit more complex, was combining the techniques of EMDR with some of my impairments from my brain injury. At times, the combination of learning specific and precise movements whilst listening or speaking was particularly difficult as my brain struggles to do more than one thing at a time. However, with a lot of learning and often emotionally challenging discussions, I was able to improve. Slowly, my nightmares reduced, and most of all my flashbacks stopped. It was such a relief to no longer be completely blindsided by these distressing experiences that often happened so unexpectedly. I also no longer felt so overwhelmingly threatened by so many things. Gradually, my heightened sense of self-protection and vulnerability lowered to a more moderate level, although it did not completely go 'back to normal'. For a long time, I had to work hard at managing my emotions, using a variety of techniques to stop the rapid escalation of stress. It took at least a year for my anxiety to lower to such a level that I began to want to try to be with people again; to go back to some of the activities that I used to enjoy. Finally, in 2023, I attempted to return to some activities – travel, going to shops, and even to have a coffee in a café with a friend.

(v) My Brain Injury is Here to Stay

Returning to the North Wales Brain Injury Service was in some ways a 'restart' of my neurorehabilitation. After years of limitations to participation and engagement due to my fear, grief and behavioural avoidance, I had finally overcome these traumatic and pandemic psychological difficulties and was ready to see if I could take an active part in normal life again. It felt like I was picking up where I had left off with the initial programme of rehab that I had started with Rudi way back in early 2020 before Covid-19 arrived and disrupted everything. The pandemic had disrupted everything, including my progression with rehabilitation, in so many ways.

My return to rehab was now about adapting to my brain injury, and developing new techniques to managing in different situations. I had some simple rehab goals. I wanted to be able to go for dinner with my partner, I wanted to try to have a coffee in a café with a friend, and I wanted to find a sustainable way to continue to work. I also wanted to return to travelling to the mountains across Europe, where I had always loved cycling and hiking. All of these goals had some similarities: the ability to manage my cognitive and sensory overload in busy social situations, how to focus on an individual conversation in a noisy place, how to make decisions in a complex environment, and how to manage my neurological fatigue.

In 2023, the World Health Organisation had declared that the pandemic was officially over. Society had now 'returned to normal' in many ways, and cafes, cinemas, shops, work places and airports had all re-opened. These places now offered ample opportunities for me to start exploring what they were like to experience with my brain injury, and how I could adapt to be able to visit them again. Supermarkets became the first experiment and slowly I developed the cognitive ability to let the constant background noise and movement of other shoppers just 'flow' past me without trying to process or respond to all this stimuli. Rehab taught me to deploy various breathing techniques, along with slowing everything down in my brain, which really helped with my slow speed of processing. This was combined with a pre-prepared shopping list to reduce the need to make decisions in the shop, which was essential given my executive dysfunction. In addition, I worked on letting go of control and developed a change of attitude to accept that it didn't matter how long it took or even if I didn't get everything. Finally, after three years of online shopping, I was able to go back to going to the supermarket. A simple, everyday activity, but it meant a lot to me, even though I usually had to rest and recover afterwards for several hours.

Other activities have proven to be much more challenging for me to do with my brain injury. In particular, going to a café or restaurant is very difficult. With my cognitive communication disorder, it is incredibly hard for me to manage to focus on listening to and speaking with the person who is sitting next to me, and I usually get completely overloaded very quickly and have to leave. I still find that my brain struggles with all the background noise and tries to pay equal attention to every other conversation in the room. It is like listening to multiple radio stations at the same time, each one interrupting the other, when you can't find a way to tune in properly to the station you actually want to listen to.

It is possible that the years of social isolation that I experienced, due to my fear of Covid-19 and post-traumatic stress, have made this sensory challenge much worse. Like an underused muscle, my brain had little experience of paying attention in busy places during the pandemic. Similar to other skills, I have now gradually come to understand that it is important to practice these cognitive functions in normal environments.

There is evidence that 'Environmental Enrichment' can have a positive impact on brain injury recovery. It is based on the concept that increased stimulation, from physical, cognitive and emotional sources, can enhance brain function – a sort of 'use it or lose it' hypothesis.

> The concept of environmental enrichment (EE) refers to exposure to and engagement with complex and stimulating environments, and there is extensive evidence that EE can beneficially influence the size, morphology and function of the brain, through synaptic modification and synaptogenesis, the shape and size of dendritic spines (or spine remodeling), axon collateral sprouting, hippocampal (dentate gyrus) neurogenesis and survival of neurons, and brain network connectivity; and such changes have been associated with improvements in functional performance.
> (Miller et al., 2013)

Even without the restrictions of the pandemic and the Covid-19 lockdowns, it has been recognised that people with a brain injury often have limited stimulation due to their difficulties in working or going out socially. One study has noted that people with a traumatic brain injury are more likely to have reduced environmental enrichment due to the limitations they experience as a result of their impairments:

> Moderate-severe TBI patients … are commonly unable to engage in the complex activities of work,

school and social activities as a result of TBI-induced decrements in cognitive, physical, perceptual and emotional functioning. These patients are especially at risk of reduced behavioral (and thereby neural) stimulation in the sub-acute and chronic stages of injury (after discharge from in-patient rehabilitation facilities), where there is often reduced environmental stimulation and/or reduced support to foster engagement in the environment.

(Miller et al., 2013)

This study goes on to note the importance of 'Environmental Enrichment' to brain capability and capacity. They found that it is possible that enhanced environmental enrichment may protect against hippocampal atrophy in the chronic stages of traumatic brain injury, and therefore help reduce the degeneration of cognitive functions.

Further research has explored the factors that can affect neuroplasticity, both in terms of activities that can help increase it and those aspects that can reduce the brain's plasticity.

Brain plasticity, also termed neuroplasticity, refers to the brain's life-long ability to reorganize itself in response to various changes in the environment, experiences, and learning. The brain is a dynamic organ capable of responding to stimulating or depriving environments, activities, and circumstances … Brain plasticity can be defined as the brain's capacity for structural and functional reorganization that depends on experience and circuit use. This capacity is heavily governed by the principle "use it or lose it" that spans from the intense "use" during development (experience-expectant plasticity) to experience-dependent plasticity in adolescence and adulthood. The capacity for neuroplasticity may be "lost" when circumstances (isolation) or physiological capacities (aging/disease) become unfavourable.

(Milbocker et al., 2024)

In my case, it is possible that my capacity for neuroplasticity was reduced by the combination of the isolation of Covid-19 and the effects of my brain injury and my subsequent reduction in capability and engagement in activities. However whilst I might have experienced limited environmental complexity over the last few years, along with increased social isolation, I did exercise every day. Research has found that exercise is significant in stimulating neuroplasticity, including both aerobic activity and resistance training.

Given my reduced social engagement and limited environmental stimuli over so many years after my accident and during the pandemic, it is unsurprising that I now still find it very difficult to go to a café, office or airport. With support from my neuropsychologist, friends, family and my partner, I am continuing to try to expand my range of 'places' and 'experiences'. This remains a learning process, and each outing offers up new challenges but also new opportunities to understand a bit more about what my brain finds difficult and overwhelming. I am developing new techniques and testing alternative approaches to manage some of these cognitive impacts, but the experimental approach can also have a negative effect on my fatigue. Overdoing things has long been part of my identity, and although I try to plan and manage my reduced capacity, I still experience frequent periods of overload and neurological fatigue. As I continue with my brain injury journey, I remind myself that rehab is a marathon not a sprint!

References

Milbocker, K. A., Smith, I. F., & Klintsova, A. Y. (2024). Maintaining a dynamic brain: A review of empirical findings describing the roles of exercise, learning, and environmental enrichment in neuroplasticity from 2017–2023. *Brain Plasticity (Amsterdam, Netherlands)*, 9(1–2), 75–95. https://doi.org/10.3233/BPL-230151

Miller, L. S., Colella, B., Mikulis, D., Maller, J., & Green, R. E. (2013). Environmental enrichment may protect against hippocampal atrophy in the chronic stages of traumatic brain injury. *Frontiers in Human Neuroscience*, 7, 506. https://doi.org/10.3389/fnhum.2013.00506

Sutton, J. (2025). 'Covid's over. Except it's not' Editorial. *The Psychologist*, Jan/Feb 25.

Chapter 6

Reflections

Sue Williams and Rudi Coetzer

Sue's Journal September 2024

Alpe D'Huez, French Alps

Steadily my feet turn the pedals as I ride up the steep long climb of Alpe d'Huez, a natural cycling rhythm that's been perfected over so many years. I breathe deeply, drawing the alpine air down into my lungs, the oxygen fuelling my muscles for the long haul. The sun beats down on my back and sweat rolls down my face. I look over my shoulder across to the towering peaks and glaciers of the Ecrin National Park, listening for the sound of the marmots on the wind. The silence and beauty of the mountains surround me. It will be a long climb up here, from the valley to the top, a sustained endurance effort that I am so used to doing on my bike. I'm in the zone, just me and the climb.

It has been a long time since I was last here. In 2016, I raced up Alpe d'Huez, the iconic cycling climb made famous by the Tour de France. Back then I was at my peak, lean, fit, and fast up hills. It was the final climb in an endurance race, 110 miles over the mountains in the French alps, with a

DOI: 10.4324/9781003509134-9

mix of snow storms and the blazing hot sun. I still remember riding up Alpe d'Huez at the end: legs exhausted, lungs straining, the road lined with cheering crowds and photographers. I had trained for years to attempt this, and I cried tears of joy and relief when I crossed the finish line at the summit. Lying in bed that night back in 2016, aching from head to foot, I felt such a wonderful glow inside. I'd done it!

Today, there are no crowds here and the road is quiet. It's out of season, mid-week in late September. It is the only climb I will manage to do today. Although I can still cycle a bit nowadays, it takes a lot out of my brain so I have to limit how much I ride. In the quietness of the Alps, settling into the familiar rhythm of the climb, it is a chance to reflect on everything that has happened over the years. So much has changed: me, my family, friends, activities, work and even wider society as a result of both my brain injury and Covid-19.

At the start of this book, I asked myself two questions. Did Covid-19 make a difference to my neurorehabilitation? Did having a traumatic brain injury affect my ability to cope with the pandemic? The simple answer to both is 'yes'. When I think back, I can see clearly now the intersection between my brain injury, trauma, and the pandemic – an unholy trinity that had significant and often overwhelming consequences for me.

In part, this was 'bad timing' – the pandemic happened whilst I was, in many ways, just starting my neurorehabilitation. In early 2020, I had only been attending rehab at the North Wales Brain Injury Service for a few months with Rudi. At this early stage, I was still at the 'understanding' point, gradually trying to learn about what was happening in my brain. I was a long way off from knowing about the extent and implications of my cognitive impairments, and even further from developing practical strategies that would enable me to adjust to a new way of living again. To have so much change in society at this point in my rehab journey meant that it was difficult to find opportunities to re-engage with activities in a slow and experimental manner. It would have been problematic to try out new strategies when everything was closed and people were unable to spend time together. Equally, the timing of the start of the pandemic meant that I had also not understood or properly processed my traumatic visceral memories from my accident. Like a powerful magnet, my psychological fear of the virus found a strong connection with my flashbacks and nightmares from my accident. The constant warning messages that filled daily life during the pandemic were a significant factor in my heightened fear and anxiety – an unintended consequence of the need for a strong societal approach to restrict behaviour at the start of the Covid-19 lockdown.

If the pandemic had started when I was further along in my rehab journey, and after I had had time and opportunity to properly process the psychological trauma of my accident, it is possible that my experience would have been different. There is significant evidence of how long 'adjustment' takes in neurorehabilitation, and to have the extensive societal change of Covid-19 at this point was probably the worst possible timing. This was compounded by the distressing loss of both my brother and mum in the same period. In the event of future significant disruptive life events, for example, another pandemic or bereavement, it is worth giving extra consideration to where someone is in the rehab process. As I found, when there is too much change happening at the same time, acceptance and adjustment becomes impossible. In a world of constantly shifting sands, the only way to find stability can often be to just hang on. In order to go forward, I needed to have a period of consistency and less drastic change in my personal life and wider society in order to build a solid foundation for future progress.

The social isolation and lack of opportunities for meaningful activities also provided fertile ground for depression and anxiety during Covid-19. This is something that affected many people during the pandemic, but the evidence shows that people with a brain injury also have a much greater likelihood of suffering from depression and anxiety. Adding family bereavement to this situation meant that it was probably inevitable that my mental health would suffer significantly. Finding ways to cope with this, especially during the various lockdown periods, emphasised the importance of combining 'psychological' as well as 'neurological' support in my brain injury rehabilitation. I very much appreciated Rudi's support during this exceptionally challenging time, and the value of having the time and opportunity to take forward a 'talking therapy' approach in my rehab sessions.

Despite all this support, there is no doubt that the societal and psychological impact of Covid-19 disrupted and delayed my rehabilitation progress. As the previous chapters have noted, after the pandemic subsided and when life began to return to some semblance of 'normal', I returned to rehab with the North Wales Brain Injury Service. I continue to work with my new neuropsychologist on developing strategies to adjust to the effects of my brain injury. As society has 're-opened' completely, I am now able to practice everyday activities like going to the cinema or a café, and even international travel again (albeit in very limited circumstances). This has had an impact on the demand for NHS rehab services, as some of us with a brain injury need longer on-going support after the restrictions of the pandemic and our rehabilitation has been somewhat delayed.

However, despite all these challenges, there have been some benefits of the societal changes arising from Covid-19, especially for someone like me with a brain injury. In particular, the shift to 'online' communication, which has made many things easier for me. I am only able to do my job as a researcher because I can work almost exclusively from home. Due to the societal shift as a result of the pandemic, the majority of my meetings and conferences now have an 'online' option. As a result, I am able to join in equally despite being unable to attend in-person due to the difficulties I have with managing busy social environments and background conversations. In addition, I have been able to join various dedicated brain injury groups and creative therapeutic classes now that so much activity is offered online. This helps me to access a much wider range of opportunities, and reduces the geographical inequalities of living in a more rural area, as well as meaning that I don't have to try to travel in order to attend. Whilst I greatly appreciate all of this online participation, I do think this does need to be combined with the benefits of spending time with people in person. I hope that as we go forward as a society, we are mindful of balancing the virtual world with the need to ensure that people with a brain injury are encouraged and supported to join in with 'real life' activities as much as possible.

Sue's Journal September, 2024
Alpe d'Huez Final Climb

As I continue to cycle up the climb, I think about who I am now. I know that I am different, both my brain injury and the psychological trauma of my accident and the pandemic have changed me forever. But Covid-19 no longer terrifies me and I have slowly learned to manage the overwhelming stress and fear that the virus used to bring. I know that my brain injury will always be part of me and it will affect my life every day, changing what I can do in ways that most people cannot see and even less comprehend. It has taken so much strength and determination to get to the point where I am today, climbing a mountain on my bike in the French Alps.

When I think about the critical attributes that are needed for neurorehabilitation, instead of 'acceptance', which always strikes me as being somewhat passive and disheartening, I think of the power of endurance and resilience, the same attributes that it takes to ride up an alpine climb. All the people I have met with a brain injury have shown incredible strength in the face of adversity. Like them, I have had to overcome much greater challenges than I had ever experienced before my brain injury. I am in it for the 'long haul', and I will need all my endurance to continue to improve and live well. I will have my brain injury for the rest of my life and I will continue to have to learn new strategies and adapt to different difficulties. Equally, life will continue to throw random curve balls, and none of us know what might be around the proverbial corner. I have learnt over the last six years that life can be distressing, complicated and confusing. Our ability to navigate our way through this complexity requires courage, insight and resilience in order to respond to unexpected change. My brain injury significantly knocked my confidence and reduced my level of psychological resilience, contributing to my inability to cope with family bereavement and the pandemic. As a result of much rehabilitation, I now feel much stronger in my sense of self. My resilience has increased and I once again have some confidence in my ability to manage life's inevitable shocks.

Most of all I have found happiness and optimism again, feelings that for so many years were beyond me. Rather than feeling 'impaired', I am now proud of my incredible brain. I recognise how hard my brain now has to work to do even some basic things, so much harder than it ever had to do before. My brain often feels that it has to sprint whilst everyone else's brain is just sauntering along, and even then I often fail to keep up; it is not that my brain is less capable, if anything, it has proven itself to be more capable in adapting and working so hard. As so many things take much more cognitive effort and my brain has to find 'work-arounds' to do the same things, it is not surprising that everything takes longer and causes immense fatigue. It is a testament to how strong my brain is that it continues to face this challenge and put such an incredible effort in, day after day. I 'feel' the cognitive strain inside my brain, sometimes trembling like a weightlifter trying to lift and hold the bar. I push myself just as hard as I used to, in fact, harder at times. However, equally difficult, has been learning the importance of not trying too hard; it takes real determination, focus and planning to hold back and rest my brain in order to keep going in the long run. The challenge of having a brain injury has been much greater than anything I had ever faced before, and I am proud of myself for continuing to climb this mountain of rehabilitation.

I could not have done this alone. My rehab journey has involved so many people, who have all supported me with such kindness and compassion. As I cycle up the last few miles of the steep climb of Alpe d'Huez, I smile to myself. Despite the empty road, I am not riding alone. I am surrounded by my 'virtual rehab peloton'. In cycling terms the peloton offers so much: team members protect you from headwinds, offer a wheel in a sprint, and pace you up a long climb. No-one rides alone, and each individual is an integral part of a wonderful whole. As I reflect on the last few years, my virtual rehab peloton is full of all the people who have helped me in so many ways. From cycling companions who have continued to make me feel a part of the club, to mountaineering friends who have taken me on hikes across the hills of Snowdonia, even carrying my rucksack in the early days. Numerous work colleagues who have helped with so many tasks, and have always left me feeling that I am still good at my job and have something to offer professionally. I will always appreciate the professional clinical support I have had from Rudi, particularly during the challenging days of Covid-19. Without his sensitive, caring and compassionate approach, along with his clinical expertise and knowledge, I would have been in a much worse place during the pandemic. As I carry on with my rehab, I am also grateful for the on-going advice of my current neuropsychologist who continues to help me find my way to living well with my brain injury.

Closer to me, is my fantastic core group of friends. I am incredibly fortunate to have so many kind, considerate and understanding people in my life, who have been there for me week in week out over the last six years. They too have had to learn a lot about my brain injury and have approached this with such sensitivity and consideration. Despite my concern about being a somewhat useless and unreliable friend as I have to frequently cancel activities due to the unpredictable nature of my neurological fatigue, they have continued to include me in their plans and encourage me to join them whenever I can. At my side, there is also my sister and oldest brother. Together we have formed a tight-knit family, at the heart of which remains my mum and youngest brother in spirit, even though they are no longer with us in person. My sister and brother continue to provide consistent support, quietly behind the scenes. Although there are probably many things they don't quite understand about my odd brain, I know without any doubt that they are always there for me, as I am for them.

There is one person missing from my 'virtual' peloton. Not because he is not important; in fact, he is the most central person in my life. Rather than just existing in my mind, he is here with me as always, cycling determinedly up this never-ending steep climb. Without Mike, my partner, my life would not be the same. No-one gives enough thought to how a brain injury affects not just the individual, but also their partner in so many ways. Neither of us expected this to happen and we have both had to learn so much about the effect of my brain injury, and cope with the impact that it has had on so many things. It has affected both our lives and from the moment my head hit the car we have both had to change. I do not have enough words to express how much he means to me, and how his love and support has enabled me to cope during the darkest days of my brain injury, the pandemic and after losing my brother and my mum. He has always been there for me, making me laugh, urging me on, holding me when my world falls apart and most of all ensuring that I do not have to face having a brain injury on my own.

I look over my shoulder and see him pushing hard up the final steep sections of the climb. We join forces for the last few metres, the summit is in sight. Legs spinning, lungs heaving, gasping, laughing. Same as we have done so many times before. We shout encouragement at each other: 'go on, go on, there's the end, give it everything'. Side by side we ride, and together we cross the finish line.

Index

For Product Safety Concerns and Information please contact our EU
representative GPSR@taylorandfrancis.com
Taylor & Francis Verlag GmbH, Kaufingerstraße 24, 80331 München, Germany

www.ingramcontent.com/pod-product-compliance
Lightning Source LLC
Chambersburg PA
CBHW051959270326
41929CB00015B/2720